DIGESTIVE DISTRESS BEGONE....

Simple menu changes combined with the right herbal tea or tincture can make a world of difference in your digestive tract. In the following pages, a knowledgeable herbalist offers natural good-for-you solutions for the most common discomforts of 20th century life:

- Colic
- Constipation
- Crohns's Disease
- Diarrhea
- Diverticulitis
- Colitis
- Gas
- Gastritis
- Heartburn
- Hemorrhoids
- Indigestion
- Irritable Bowel Syndrome
- Ulcers

About the Author

CJ Puotinen has studied with some of America's leading herbalists and is a member of the Herb Research Foundation, the American Herb Association and the Northeast Herbal Association. In addition to magazine and journal articles on health and medicinal herbs, she is the author of *Herbal Teas, Nature's Antiseptics: Tea Tree Oil and Grapefruit Seed Extract,* and *Herbs to Help You Breathe Freely,* all published by Keats Publishing, Inc.

A KEATS GOOD HERB GUIDE

MEDICINE for the 21st CENTURY

HERBS TO IMPROVE DIGESTION

Herbal remedies for stomach pain, constipation, ulcers, colitis and other gastrointestinal problems

CJ Puotinen

Keats Publishing, Inc. 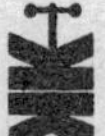 New Canaan, Connecticut

Herbs to Improve Digestion is intended solely for informational and educational purposes, and not as medical advice. Please consult a medical or health professional if you have questions about your health.

HERBS TO IMPROVE DIGESTION

Library of Congress Cataloging-in-Publication Data

Puotinen, CJ
Herbs to improve digestion / CJ Puotinen.
p. cm.
Includes bibliographical references and index.
ISBN 0-87983-742-X
1. Indigestion—Diet therapy. 2. Herbs—Therapeutic use.
I. Title.
RC827.P88 1996
616.3'0654—dc20 96-24279
CIP

Printed in the United States of America

Published by Keats Publishing, Inc.
27 Pine Street (Box 876)
New Canaan, Connecticut 06840-0876

98 97 96 6 5 4 3 2 1

CONTENTS

INTRODUCTION

Heartburn, indigestion, gas, constipation, ulcers, diarrhea, intestinal disorders, irritable bowel syndrome, colitis, stomach cancer, colon cancer, leaky gut syndrome, hemorrhoids, spastic colon, stomach cramps and diverticulitis are so common in America today that anyone judging by television commercials or hospital admission records would assume they're inevitable. Everyone has them.

Not so. Until this century in the United States, hardly anyone did, and even today in many parts of the world, these chronic disorders are unheard of. Digestive distress is a product of modern civilization.

Orthodox physicians treat symptoms, not causes. That's what allopathic (symptom-oriented) medicine is all about. But suppressing symptoms doesn't address the cause of a problem, which is why people who treat their heartburn with antacids, their ulcer symptoms with prescription drugs, or their constipation with laxatives are seldom cured. To cure an illness, you must remove its cause.

The cause of nearly every digestive ailment in modern America is our diet, which is low in fiber, high in fat and cholesterol, high in refined sugars and flours, depleted in nutrients, preserved with chemicals, enhanced with artificial flavors and swallowed with beverages containing ingredients no one can pronounce. Of course, it doesn't help that we breathe polluted air, drink contaminated water, fill our lives with stress, get far too little exercise and eat on the run. It's a wonder we don't *all* have ulcers, not to mention heart disease, cancer and diabetes.

It doesn't have to be that way. Simple menu changes combined with the right herbal teas and tinctures can make a world of digestive difference. Herbs are not magical drugs.

If you live on doughnuts, French fries and microwaved hamburgers, no herbal tea can give you glowing good health. In combination with an improved diet, however, the world of herbs offers lasting support to every cell and organ in the body.

THE DIGESTIVE PROCESS

Under normal conditions, digestion is an efficient process that transforms food into energy, nutrients and waste products, all of which are sent to appropriate parts of the body for dispersal and disposal. The food is acted upon by chemicals, such as the stomach's hydrochloric acid, and enzymes. Digestion begins in the mouth with saliva, which, under optimum conditions, is well-blended with food during chewing. Enzymes combine with moisture to transform carbohydrates into maltose, an energy-producing sugar. Well chewed and with its carbohydrates predigested, the food travels down the esophagus to the stomach, where it encounters, among other things, the enzymes rennin, pepsin and lipase, which digest milk, protein and fats. Hydrochloric acid breaks down proteins and the fiber of vegetables, releasing nutrients, destroying bacteria and regulating the body's acid-alkaline balance. Food then travels to the small intestine, where it encounters bile, pancreatic lipase, tripsin, lactase, amylopsin and other enzymes. Altogether, the body uses over 600 enzymes, each of which performs a separate function in the body. Without them, we cannot convert food into energy or extract its nutrients; in fact, without them none of our bodies' processes would function properly.

The liver, which lies beside the stomach just below the rib cage, has two important functions. It separates toxins from the blood stream, protecting the body from poisons, and it produces bile, a powerful digestive chemical, which it sends to the gallbladder for injection into the small intestine. We associate the stomach with digestion, but the liver, our largest and busiest organ, is even more important. People can survive without stomachs but no one survives without a liver.

The "small" in its name makes the small intestine sound insignificant, but this is where digestion really takes place. Food broken down by hydrochloric acid and stomach enzymes is completely transformed during its journey through this 23-foot tube by bile from the gallbladder and enzymes from the pancreas, releasing most of its nutrients to the intestine's blood-rich lining. What's left exits into the large intestine.

The large intestine absorbs water, excretes mucus and (under normal conditions) hosts large numbers of beneficial bacteria which complete the digestive process by absorbing some nutrients and releasing others. As food residue travels through the large intestine and its water is absorbed, it becomes more compact and is eventually expelled. When the diet is rich in fiber, the resulting stool is large, soft and easy to eliminate, taking harmful bacteria, toxins and other waste material with it.

Evolution and the Human Digestive Tract

Anthropologists tell us that human beings have been evolving for 4 million years. Even if theories of more recent evolution are correct, placing today's humans on the planet for only 50,000 to 75,000 years, it's obvious that our species evolved on a diet very different from our own. The first significant shift in human diet followed the agricultural revolution, when people domesticated plants, then animals. For the first time, a stable and reliable supply of food could be grown in one place, gradually shifting us from the truly omnivorous fare of nomadic hunter/gatherers, who had no choice but to eat whatever the earth provided, to the more selective diet of a settled people who produced more than they could eat. This made it possible to stay in one place and, even more important, to prevent starvation by setting the surplus aside for future use. Because grains store well, farmers developed effective methods for growing them and they became a staple food. Some nutritionists believe that the human digestive tract is still adapting to this cultural change, which took place only 10,000 years ago.

Even after humans began baking bread and roasting a more stable supply of meat, they consumed most of their food raw or only partly cooked and they still consumed a variety of foods—whatever could be collected from the sea, rivers, lakes or land. Grains were ground whole, never stripped of their bran to make white rice or flour. Vegetables were eaten raw or lightly cooked; they weren't deep-fried, cooked in a pressure cooker, canned, irradiated or microwaved. Salting (in whole, unprocessed sea or mined salt), fermentation (yogurt, sauerkraut, cheese, wine, beer and pickles) and drying were the only means of preserving perishable foods beyond their harvest. Sugar as we know it didn't exist, sweets like raw honey were rare treats and salt was never refined to separate its trace minerals for sale to industry. No one used pesticides, herbicides, preservatives, chemical additives, artificial flavors, flavor enhancers, chemical sweeteners or artificial fats. No one drank pasteurized milk, pasteurized juice or carbonated colas. Even cave men, who in our popular imagination lived on fresh-killed meat, didn't eat it every day. It is only in the last 150 years in the industrial West, especially the last 50 years in North America, that traditional foods have been replaced by substances human digestive organs were never before exposed to. Fifty years of technology in 4 million years of digestive evolution is like 1 second in a 24-hour day. We've been eating modern fare for the blink of an eye.

In the 1920s and '30s, Dr. Weston Price, a California dentist, and his wife traveled the world in search of cultures that had little or no contact with the industrial West. In every case, adherence to a traditional diet of unrefined food meant freedom from disease while exposure to "civilization" (refined flour, sugar and canned foods) brought with it dental cavities, jaw deformities, crooked teeth and all the illnesses we think of as "normal," including digestive complaints.

Nutrition and Physical Degeneration the book that chronicles Price's findings, has become a classic.

The Raw and the Cooked

Of all its enemies, the single factor that has most disrupted normal digestion is heat, the process of cooking. Temperatures above 112 to 120 degrees Fahrenheit (44 to 49 degrees Centigrade) destroy key nutrients and enzymes in food, transforming it from "live" to "dead." Raw or live food contains all its enzymes, vitamins, minerals, volatile essential oils, plant hormones, bioflavonoids, chlorophyll and other pigments, natural disinfectants and infection fighters, fiber and other nutrients. Our species evolved on a live diet of fruits, berries, roots, vegetables and other raw fare, and those are the foods a healthy body digests most easily.

Experiments with the healing effects of raw food are practically unknown in the United States, but the biological clinics of Europe have repeatedly shown that raw foods cure disease. In Scandinavia, Switzerland, Germany, Austria and other countries, physicians treat cancer and every other illness with raw foods, herbs and other natural therapies. Reports of their success and of related laboratory research and clinical trials are widely published in medical and scientific journals. Although you're not likely to hear this advice from American physicians, you may do more for your colitis, diverticulitis, ulcers, constipation, hemorrhoids, irritable bowel syndrome, Crohn's disease, hepatitis, spastic colon, gallstones, liver disease, chronic diarrhea, gastritis or heartburn with raw food and herbs than with any prescription drugs or surgery.

The Diet Debates

If you begin exploring raw food regimes, you'll see that menu planning inspires passionate debate. Some think fruits are the worst thing you can eat. Others, called fruitarians, believe that humans are meant to live on raw fruit and nothing else. Fletcherites, disciples of Horace Fletcher, who developed a nutritional healing system in the 19th century, chewed every bite of food for 10 to 15 minutes. Ehretists, disciples of Arnold Ehret, still follow his mucus-less diet and avoid mucus-causing foods. Advocates of food-combining believe that fruits should be eaten alone and early in the day because the body digests them faster than other foods; protein and starches should never be eaten together; protein should be eaten alone or with leafy green vegetables; and other vegetables should be eaten alone or with grains or legumes. This strategy is followed by both raw foodists, such as Ann Wigmore's followers, and those who eat cooked foods as well. Harvey and Marilyn Diamond's *Fit for Life* was a national best seller and helped make food combining a household word. Other approaches to nutrition involve:

- Monitoring pH levels of urine and saliva in order to adjust the diet for proper pH balance.
- Eating chlorella or spirulina or blue-green algae.
- Following a hypoglycemic diet plan of numerous small meals throughout the day, or
- Eating a macrobiotic diet.

There is no shortage of unusual theories about diet, and every one of them works for someone. The important thing is to find a diet that works for you.

The Importance of Juicing

While it's true that Americans don't eat enough fiber, an impaired digestive tract may not be able to cope with a sudden supply of raw produce. Juicing is a popular therapy because juices are concentrated, nutritious and easy to assimilate. They are, in a sense, predigested. Someone whose stomach and intestines would be overwhelmed by even a few raw carrots can absorb the nutrients in five pounds of carrots just by swallowing their juice. Fresh juices contain all of the enzymes and nutrients found in the fruits or vegetables that made them.

Once you have a juicer and a good supply of produce, preferably organically grown, you can experiment with juice fasting (going without solid food while drinking only juice and water or tea for several days or weeks). Juice fasting is a popular way to treat digestive disorders because it lets overworked organs rest while improving the body's absorption of nutrients. A gradual return to solid food and appropriate menu planning completes the cure.

Looking for a juice that treats colic? Pharmacist William Lee, Ph.D., recommends 10 ounces of carrot juice mixed with 6 ounces of spinach juice; or a blend of 3 ounces of beet juice, 3 ounces of cucumber juice and 10 ounces of carrot juice. For colitis, he prescribes papaya juice by itself, carrot and spinach juices, apple and carrot or a blend of beet, carrot and cucumber. The herbalist John Lust recommends cabbage juice for peptic ulcers, carrot juice for gallstones and a blend of carrot, celery and parsley juices for indigestion. And for every digestive ailment, Ann Wigmore recommended wheat grass or barley grass juice. Grass juice, by the way, is very concentrated and a powerful cleanser. Before embarking on wheat grass or barley grass therapy, read Wigmore and other authorities, then start slowly.

FOOD SENSITIVITIES

A true omnivore eats everything: a variety of seeds, nuts, fruits, vegetables, meats, eggs, roots and tubers—anything and everything that's edible.

Most Americans, on the other hand, eat the same things every day. We may think we're eating a variety of foods, but in most cases it's just different versions of wheat, eggs, milk, potatoes and beef. A breakfast of eggs, sausage, milk, white toast and hash browns is the same as a lunch of hamburger, milkshake, white bun and fries, which is the same as a dinner of pizza, steak and potatoes or white pasta with ice cream. These meals, which are typical for adults and children across the country, are devoid of fruits and vegetables, low in enzymes, fiber and nutrients, high in fat, calories and toxins, and likely to generate food sensitivities.

Rainbow Meal Plan

What's an example of variety? Bruce Pacetti, a dentist and nutritionist, refined the discoveries of Weston Price, the anthropologist-dentist. Pacetti found that many patients with chronic health problems, including the overgrowth of the intestinal yeast, *Candida albicans*, suffered from food sensitivities. To provide for better digestion and a wider range of nutrients while reducing allergic reactions, he developed the Rainbow Meal Plan. Each meal consists of one small serving from each of the following food groups:

- Complete protein (meat, fish, poultry, eggs)
- Legumes and grains (beans, whole grains)
- Root vegetables (carrots, beets, Jerusalem artichokes, onions)
- Yellow or white vegetables (corn, cucumbers, parsnips, turnips, squash)
- Green vegetables (artichokes, asparagus, broccoli, leeks, peas)
- Red/orange/purple vegetables (beets, carrots, pumpkin, red cabbage, red peppers, sweet potatoes, tomatoes)
- Leafy green vegetables (collard greens, endive, kale, lettuce, mustard greens, parsley).

There are no dairy products, fruits or sweeteners in this diet plan, yet it provides abundant vitamins, fiber and nutrients. Pacetti encouraged his patients to eat as many meals per day as they wanted, having six different foods, one from each group, per meal. This color-based plan for nutritional variety offers health benefits to everyone, not just those with candidiasis. Vegetarians can adapt the plan by eliminating the first category, and anyone wanting to increase variety in menu planning can use it for inspiration. The Rainbow Meal Plan is explained in detail in *The Candida Albicans Yeast-Free Cookbook* by Pat Connolly and Associates of the Price-Pottenger Nutrition Foundation

Food Intolerences

Physicians who study food sensitivities say the most common offenders are milk and wheat. These are the foods we eat most often, and the body builds up an intolerance for them. A simple way to treat irritable bowel syndrome, diverticulitis, gastritis, flatulence, Crohn's disease, ulcerative colitis and other digestive disorders is to stay away from all milk products and all wheat products for a month. In many cases, the condition improves quickly.

The most extreme wheat intolerance is celiac sprue or celiac disease, a chronic disorder of the small intestine caused by sensitivity to gluten, a protein found not only in wheat but in rye, oats and barley. This disorder interferes with the body's absorption of fat, protein, carbohydrates, iron, water and vitamins A, D, E and K. Caused by a hereditary defect and found mostly in people of northwestern European ancestry, celiac sprue is far more common in Ireland than in the U.S. Symptoms usually begin in childhood with the introduction of wheat cereal or other foods containing gluten. They include painful bloating, stunted growth, iron-deficiency anemia, bone deformation and pale, bulky, malodorous stools. In some cases, symptoms disappear during adolescence and reappear in adulthood. The only successful treatment for celiac sprue is the careful avoidance of all foods containing gluten; most doctors prescribe a high protein, low fat diet with vitamin supplementation.

The milk story in any examination of food sensitivities is complicated by a far more widespread inability to digest milk. If you consume cream, milk, cheese, cream cheese, cottage cheese, ice cream, ice milk, sour cream, frozen yogurt, whey or products containing nonfat milk solids and within an hour feel gassy and uncomfortable, your body is probably unable to produce lactase, the enzyme that digests lactose, the sugar in milk.

One solution is to use Lactaid, a lactase enzyme supplement from AkPharma, Inc. Lactaid tablets can be taken when eating or drinking any dairy product; liquid Lactaid can be added to milk a day before drinking it. Another solution is to eat freshly prepared yogurt or a similar cultured milk dish for its bacterial fermentation predigests milk sugars.

However, supplemental enzymes and friendly bacteria cannot protect against adverse reactions to milk if they result from something other than insufficient lactase. Some who are fond of dairy products have experimented with goat's milk cheese or yogurt, for goat's milk contains less lactose than cow's milk. Others have left milk entirely and now use soy milk, almond milk and other substitutes. The demand for dairy-free "dairy" products has spawned a fast-growing health food industry of soy- or nut-based milk substitutes and nondairy ice cream, coffee creamers, yogurt and cheese.

There is much debate and confusion over the term "food

allergy." To orthodox physicians, an allergic reaction is immediate and dramatic, like anaphylactic shock, which can be fatal, or a sudden eruption of hives. The term "food sensitivity" was coined to describe more subtle reactions that are still debilitating.

Although there are blood tests and patch tests designed to detect food allergies and sensitivities, you can conduct your own effective test at home with pencil in hand. Keep a notebook of everything you eat, when you eat it, how your body responds and how you feel. Sometimes this simple exercise will bring to light an obvious connection between cause and symptom.

Rotation Diet

A more rigorous test is the four-day rotation diet. Because it takes four days for the body to remove all traces of the foods you consume, this system schedules four days of menus according to related food groups. On Day One you might eat wheat, then no wheat at all on Days Two, Three and Four. Here is an example of four days' food groups.

Day One	Day Two	Day Three	Day Four
apples	oranges	bananas	pears
wheat	oats	rye	buckwheat
cashews	almonds	pecans	walnuts
cow's milk	almond milk	goat milk	soy milk
beef	chicken	fish	lamb
carrots	celery	radishes	parsnips
wheat bran	oat bran	rice bran	psyllium husks

On Day One, eat any bread containing wheat by itself (no multi-grain bread), any cow's milk or dairy product (cheese, cottage cheese, yogurt, etc.), any amount of apples and carrots, beef, cashew nuts, and whatever else you decide to add to the list, as long as it doesn't conflict with the next three days' foods. If your bread contains sesame seed, add it to the list so you won't eat sesame seeds again. If you have pizza for dinner (wheat and cheese) list the tomatoes, mushrooms, olive oil and anchovies you consume.

On Day Two, limit yourself to foods you did not eat the day before and will not eat again for four days. Eggs, a chicken product, can be eaten this day but not on Days One, Three or Four.

The four-day rotation diet is time-consuming and requires careful planning. You have to read labels constantly, and it's just about impossible to dine out unless you avoid sauces and salad dressings, check ingredients with your waiter or hostess and write everything down as you consume it. Unless you can verify their food sources and other ingredients, you have to stop taking vitamins and food supplements. Beverages can cause all kinds of complications. Forget Coke and Pepsi. Nearly all "healthy" soft drinks, bottled iced tea and bottled juice blends contain high-fructose corn syrup. If they contain sugar, is it from beets or sugar cane? Beer contains barley, malt, hops and yeast, and that's if you buy a German beer or a brand that lists its ingredients. American beers are notorious for containing sudsing agents, artificial colors, preservatives and chemical additives that never appear on labels. No wonder beer and pizza give you heartburn!

After you've followed this regimen for a week, start rearranging the foods. Separate wheat from beef, for example, or soy milk from walnuts. Keep food families in mind. On the day you drink soy milk, you can eat tofu, tempeh, soy sauce, miso and any other soy product. On the next three days, you have to avoid all soy foods. On the day you eat tomatoes, eat all you want of eggplant, peppers and potatoes, for all are members of the nightshade family—then avoid eating any of these "cousin" foods for four days. Tobacco, by the way, is another nightshade.

Pulse Check

Another way to test for food sensitivities is by taking your pulse. This simple procedure was discovered fifty years ago by Arthur M. Coca, M.D. Coca's discovery was simplicity itself. If you eat a food that agrees with you, your pulse rate will remain stable. If you eat one that doesn't, your pulse will increase. In his medical practice and through his book *The Pulse Test*, Dr. Coca trained thousands to monitor their diets and make their own accurate diagnoses.

In order to take the pulse test accurately, you must stop smoking for the duration of the test and be free of conditions that might disrupt your pulse, such as fighting off a cold or being sunburned.

Count your pulse for 60 seconds just after waking in the morning and just before going to bed at night. In addition, take your pulse just before each meal and again 30 minutes, 60 minutes and 90 minutes after the meal ends. Always take your pulse sitting up, except when you first wake in the morning.

Keep a food journal for two or three days, noting everything you eat at each meal and the day's pulse rates. Some connections may be obvious at once. If your pulse jumps from 65 beats per minute just before breakfast to 85 beats per minute after, something in the French toast may not agree with you. One woman discovered that her pulse raced every morning, just after she got up. After three days, she realized that the problem was her toothpaste. When she changed brands, her chronic migraine headaches disappeared.

You can use the pulse test to check individual foods and narrow your findings to a single offender. Eliminate the foods that cause your pulse to race and you'll eliminate health problems with them.

Antacids, Hydrochloric Acid and Aging

The high-fat, low-fiber, nutrient-depleted American diet sustains life; we'd all be dead if it didn't. The fact that it doesn't enhance health isn't obvious, though, or more people would stop eating it. Dietary habits are set in youth, when the body has an abundance of its own enzymes to compensate for the lack of live enzymes in food, when it has abundant gastric juices and a strong, working liver, when minor deficiencies aren't so obvious.

Things change in middle age. This is when colon cancer and diverticulitis tend to manifest, along with other illnesses that result from a lifetime of incorrect eating. As the body ages, it produces less hydrochloric acid, leading to indigestion and an inability to absorb nutrients. Hydrochloric acid is a powerful chemical that breaks down food fibers and destroys harmful bacteria. It's an important factor in preventing disease. But when the body produces less hydrochloric acid, most people misinterpret the results, believing that their indigestion and discomfort are due to too much stomach acid. When they take antacids, they further suppress the stomach's ability to generate hydrochloric acid, which makes the problem worse. An insufficient supply of hydrochloric acid interferes with digestion and leaves one more vulnerable to bacterial, viral or microbial infections.

Instead of taking antacids, you may improve by taking hydrochloric acid. HCl supplements are sold in health food stores and pharmacies. In his *Prescription for Nutritional Healing,* James Balch, M.D. suggested the following method for determining whether you need additional HCl. "Take a tablespoon of apple cider vinegar or lemon juice. If this makes your heartburn go away, then you need more stomach acid. If it makes your symptoms worse, then you have too much HCl and shouldn't take any enzyme products that contain HCl." If you don't have chronic heartburn but have occasional bouts of indigestion, try taking one HCl supplement with or slightly before a large meal. If it helps, continue adding it; if it gives you heartburn, stop.

DIGESTIVE ENZYMES

Unless you eat everything raw and everything you eat comes from farmland rich in minerals, and it's all organically grown, you probably need assistance.

Digestive enzyme products contain one, a few or many different enzymes. Most include protease, which helps digest protein; amylase, a saliva enzyme that breaks down carbohydrates; and lipase, an upper digestive tract enzyme that breaks down fats. Some brands include hydrochloric acid (HCl), pepsin, ox bile, pancreatic substances, papain, cellulose enzymes or bromelain from pineapples. Digestive enzymes are sold as powders to sprinkle on food or as tablets and capsules. There are dozens on the market, including vegetarian formulas, special blends and products for dogs and cats. Whenever you eat cooked or processed food, especially as you grow older, consider taking an enzyme supplement.

One single-ingredient, special-purpose enzyme product is Beano, which makes beans and bean products easier to digest, helping to prevent flatulence. Liquid Beano, a pet version named Curtail and bean-shaped Beano capsules are designed to be taken with the first bite of an offending food. Beano is sold by AkPharma, Inc., the makers of Lactaid, the lactase enzyme that digests milk sugars. Beano doesn't work for everyone, so experiment with small doses of offending foods. Other strategies for making beans easier to digest include sprouting them first (soak overnight in a wide-mouth jar, then drain and leave at room temperature for 24 to 36 hours), changing the cooking water once or twice (the hard-to-digest components are water-soluble) and adding savory or bay leaves to the pot during cooking. Always remove bay leaves before serving; swallowed leaves have caused internal injury.

DYING OF THIRST?

Perhaps the simplest therapy recommended for digestive problems is water. In his book *Your Body's Many Cries for Water,* F. Batmanghelidj, M.D., explained that most illness is caused not by pathogens or immune disorders, but by dehydration. "You're not sick," he declares, "you're thirsty." Plain drinking water consumed in sufficient quantity throughout the day helps prevent many health problems.

"Dyspeptic pain," wrote Dr. Batmanghelidj, "is the most important signal for the human body. It denotes dehydration. It is a thirst signal and can occur in the very young as well as in older people. Of dyspeptic pains, that of gastritis, duodenitis and heartburn should be treated with an increase in water intake alone. When there is associated ulceration, attention to the daily diet to enhance the rate of repair of the ulcer site becomes necessary."

Using water, typically one to three 8-ounce glasses at 15-minute or 1-hour intervals, Dr. Batmanghelidj has treated over 3,000 patients with dyspeptic pain who had symptoms of specific digestive diseases, such as diverticulitis, peptic ulcer or irritable bowel syndrome. In most cases, pain disappeared within eight to twenty minutes. In one case the patient, a young man, was semiconscious from ulcer pain which three doses of a prescription drug and a bottle of antacid had not relieved. His groaning misery had lasted for ten hours when Batmanghelidj dosed him with one glass of water, then, 15 minutes later, two more. Within 20 minutes he was standing, conducting normal conversations and completely free of pain.

Dr. Batmanghelidj's report on treating dyspeptic pain with water was published in the June 1993 *Journal of Clinical Gastroenterology* and several physicians have recommended his methods in their health newsletters. Dehydration is a serious consideration in treating any digestive or intestinal disorder. As Dr. Batmanghelidj cautions, other fluids like coffee and colas don't count; you should drink plain room-temperature water, up to a gallon a day with a pinch of salt added, for best results. This treatment has been successfully used to relieve migraine headaches, back pain, allergies, stress and other ailments as well.

No discussion of water would be complete without a caution regarding American tap water, which has received much negative publicity in recent years. Concerns over water safety have made bottled spring water a growth industry along with home water filters and distillers. Whatever you can do to improve the quality of the water you drink will help improve your digestion.

Reconsidering Salt

Americans are so used to hearing physicians' warnings against salt that Dr. Batmanghelidj's advice to add a pinch of salt to drinking water sounds strange at first. But he's right. While refined table salt causes serious problems, natural salt improves every body function.

All popular brands of table salt have been bleached, then treated with stabilizing agents and dehydrating chemicals. Whether coarse or finely ground, this salt is between 98- and 99-percent pure sodium chloride (NaCl), and it was dried at temperatures high enough to change its crystalline structure. Its structural changes, nutrient-stripping and added chemicals make table salt difficult for the body to assimilate, contributing to electrolyte imbalances, trace mineral deficiencies and digestive problems. The sodium content of nearly every processed food derives from refined salt.

Unfortunately, most sea salt is as processed as table salt and contains added chemicals as well. Nearly all are 98- to

99-percent pure sodium chloride and, like table salt, contain no trace minerals, only the residue of processing chemicals. Ask about these products at your health store: Real Salt, Lima Salt and Celtic Salt.

Avoiding Sugar

In nutritional circles, no one has anything good to say about white sugar and only a few defend honey, brown rice syrup, barley malt, maple syrup, dehydrated sugar cane juice or molasses. In fact, some condemn dried fruit, fruit juices and any fruit sweeter than a cranberry.

Dr. Melvin Page was one of the first to take this position. A dentist and colleague of Weston Price, Page studied Price's research and applied the findings to his patients. Through laboratory analyses, he discovered that when patients ate sugar or refined carbohydrates, their blood chemistries changed. Page recommended that anyone recovering from illness avoid all fruits and sugars; during healthy times, he recommended fruits and sweets only occasionally.

Sugar disrupts digestion by overworking the pancreas, which produces insulin, the hormone that regulates our utilization of glucose (sugar) and carbohydrates. Excessive insulin, especially in overweight people, is associated with fluid retention, sleep disorders, the production of the "bad" cholesterol LDL, low metabolism, thyroid disorders, hypoglycemia and food cravings. Internal parasites love sugar. So do *Candida albicans* yeast cells.

High fructose corn syrup is of growing concern because recent studies have shown that large quantities of high-fructose sweeteners can lead to chromium deficiency, which is associated with heart disease and diabetes.

In our culture sugar is very hard to avoid and it's addictive, but reducing or eliminating sugar from the diet often improves digestion, increases energy and improves overall health.

BENEFICIAL BACTERIA

If you live in America, the odds are you have taken antibiotics. These powerful and overused drugs take a toll: In addition to their other side effects, they destroy the beneficial intestinal bacteria we are born with. Healthy intestinal microflora typically contains between 400 and 500 different species of bacteria, most of them in the colon. An important survival mechanism, these bacteria:

- Produce enzymes
- Improve digestion
- Lower the risk of irritable bowel syndrome
- Boost the immune system
- Inhibit the growth of pathogens
- Prevent diarrhea
- Synthesize vitamins
- Detoxify the body, and
- Protect against toxins.

Because antibiotics destroy beneficial as well as harmful bacteria, antibiotic treatment often brings gastrointestinal discomfort, diarrhea, incomplete digestion, a susceptibility to yeast or fungal infections and lowered immunity.

To invite beneficial bacteria back into your system:

1. Buy acidophilus powders or supplements from your health food store's refrigerator (look for amber glass jars with distant expiration dates) and sprinkle it on food or take before breakfast, when stomach acid is less concentrated, or just after a meal, when food acts

as a buffer. Some acidophilus capsules and tablets are designed to break down later in the digestive process, and a few brands claim to survive stomach acid. *Bifidus* strains are native to humans and will reproduce in the intestines over time. Read labels carefully.

2. Use purchased yogurt, acidophilus powder or yogurt starter to make your own yogurt at home, using soy milk if desired.
3. Feed your friendly bacteria. They thrive on whey (even lactose-intolerant people can benefit from a daily tablespoon of Molkosan, a Swiss whey concentrate which does not contain milk solids), and from naturally fermented foods rich in lactic acid, such as sauerkraut and unheated, unpasteurized pickles. Onions and cabbage are reported to be good for these friendly microbes, as are dextrose, a sugar found in rice and corn, and Jerusalem artichokes. Also called sunchokes, these last are not artichokes at all but sunflowers. Their underground tubers contain inulin, a favorite food of lactobacteria. Popular in Japan as a food for intestinal health, Jerusalem artichoke flour is available in U.S. health food stores and the raw tubers are sold in many supermarkets.

THE ROLE OF EXERCISE

Two people eat the same foods, drink the same water and take the same supplements. One enjoys long walks with his dog, goes dancing every night and practices yoga. The other sits at a computer all day and watches TV all night. Which has constipation?

In addition to eating all the wrong things, Americans are alarmingly underexercised. An active lifestyle does more than improve circulation and help you lose weight; it improves digestion and elimination. Fresh air and aerobic activity are obvious prescriptions for improved digestive health, but did you know that inverted postures are just as important? Yoga offers several upside-down positions, all of which are known for their digestive benefits, but even reclining at a slight angle on a slant board for five to ten minutes a day has helped many people improve regularity without laxatives and enjoy favorite foods without after-dinner discomfort.

HERBS TO THE RESCUE!

In addition to all of the preceding strategies, you have a wealth of digestive friends in the world of herbs. Herbal medicine offers safe, effective treatments for every digestive disturbance and has stood the test of time for hundreds, if not thousands, of years.

Herbs can be eaten raw in salads, juiced with vegetables, added to soups and other foods, brewed as teas, taken in capsules and made into tinctures or liquid extracts.

Teas

The most familiar herbal preparations are teas. Teas are either infusions, made by pouring boiling water over fresh or dried leaves or blossoms; or decoctions, made by simmering roots or bark. In either case, a beverage-strength tea is made by combining 1 teaspoon dry tea (or 1 tablespoon fresh herb) with 1 cup water. Double or triple the amount of herb for a medicinal strength tea. For best results, prepare infusions in a glass or ceramic pot with a tight-fitting lid; prepare decoctions in a covered saucepan. Let infusions stand 10 to 15 minutes before straining and serving; let decoctions simmer on low heat after reaching the boiling point for 10 to 15 minutes, then let stand another 5 to 10 minutes before serving.

In some cases a cold infusion is recommended. Mix shredded or chopped plant material with cold water and let stand overnight, or place plant material in a roomy muslin bag, suspend the bag at the top of a glass jar filled with cold water and close the jar. When heavy plant matter falls to the bottom of the jar, a gentle current lifts water to the surface, where it combines again with the plant material, setting up slow percolation.

Tinctures

A tincture is a liquid extract made by soaking fresh or dried herbs in grain alcohol, such as rum or vodka, vegetable glycerine or a combination of both. Tinctures have a long shelf life and are very concentrated. However, they aren't as concentrated as their labels suggest. According to Rosemary Gladstar, who pioneered popular herbology in the 1960s and is now one of America's foremost herbalists, the minuscule doses on most tincture bottles date back to the early days of commercial tincture making when the only comparable products were homeopathic. In homeopathy, doses are measured by the drop. For lack of a better system of dosages, herbalists used similar measurements. In most cases, Gladstar asserts, when a tincture bottle recommends 15 to 20 drops, you'll do better to take half a teaspoon or even a tablespoon of tincture, depending on the herbs involved and the condition you're treating. Keep this in mind if you ever find an herbal tincture ineffective. It may be that the herb is working just fine, it's the dosage that isn't.

For information on tincture making, see the instructions for making Swedish bitters on page 56 and comfrey tincture on page 40.

Capsules

Capsules contain cut and sifted, crushed or powdered herbs. Because powdered herbs lose their potency when exposed to heat, light or humidity, they should be purchased from a reliable source and stored carefully. Kitchen cabinets near the stove are not a good place to store medicinal herbs, whether teas or capsules.

One way to insure quality capsules is to obtain high-grade

dried herbs, grind them yourself in any coffee or spice grinder and fill your own. Two-part gelatin capsules (including vegetarian capsules) come in three sizes, as do hand-operated capping devices that make filling them easy work. Some herb companies will blend and grind herbs and place them in capsules for you, and health food stores carry an increasing variety of herbal capsules.

Types of Digestive Herbs

There are literally hundreds of herbs that benefit digestion. Some stimulate gastric secretions, others increase the muscular contractions that transport food, increase the flow of saliva, relieve gas and flatulence, eliminate parasites, tone the liver or repair damaged or irritated stomach lining. Here are some of the most effective and popular herbs in 11 digestive categories.

ANTHELMINTIC: Herb that destroys or expels intestinal worms and parasites. Same as **Vermifuge** or **Parisiticide**. Examples: black walnut husk, chaparral, cloves, garlic, grapefruit seed extract, white rind of pomegranate, wormwood.

ANTIBILIOUS: Herb that combats nausea, abdominal discomfort, headache, constipation and gas caused by excessive secretions of bile. Examples: cayenne pepper, cloves, dandelion, dill, fennel, ginger, goldenseal, lavender, wormwood.

ANTIMICROBIAL: Herb that helps the body destroy or resist pathogenic micro-organisms. Examples: cloves, echinacea, eucalyptus, grapefruit seed extract, myrrh, wormwood. These are sometimes labeled antibiotic herbs.

ANTISPASMODIC: Herb that relieves or prevents involuntary muscle spasm or cramps. Examples: chamomile, cramp bark, skullcap, valerian.

ASTRINGENT: Herb that causes local contraction of the skin, blood vessels and other tissues, arresting the discharge of blood or mucus and relieving diarrhea. Most astringents contain tannin. Examples: bayberry bark, witch hazel bark, wild oak bark, uva ursi, cranesbill.

BITTER: Herb with a sharp, bitter taste that stimulates the digestive system through a reflex via the taste buds. Examples: centaury, gentian, horehound, wormwood.

CARMINATIVE: Aromatic herb containing volatile oils that stimulate peristalsis, relax the stomach, relieve intestinal cramping, help prevent gas from forming in the intestines and also help expel it. Examples: allspice, angelica, aniseed, basil, caraway, cardamom, calamus, cayenne, celery seed, chamomile, cinnamon, cloves, dill seed, fennel seed, ginger, nutmeg, peppermint.

DEMULCENT: Herb that has mucilaginous properties that soothe and protect irritated or inflamed surfaces and tissues. Important in formulas. Many are also antacids. Examples: agar agar, aloe vera gel, comfrey, fenugreek seed, flaxseed, Iceland moss, Irish moss, licorice root, mallow, marshmallow, oatmeal, psyllium husk powder, slippery elm bark.

HEPATIC: Herb that promotes the well-being of the liver and increases the secretion of bile. Liver tonic. Examples: agrimony, dandelion, goldenseal, wahoo, wild yam root, yellow dock.

LAXATIVE: Herb that promotes evacuation of the bowels. Laxatives are more gentle than cathartics, purgatives or drastics, which cause violent evacuation. Laxatives are best used in small doses or infrequently. Examples: cascara sagrada, flaxseed, senna, rhubarb root.

SIALAGOGUE: Herb that promotes the flow of saliva and aids digestion. Examples: black pepper, cayenne pepper, gentian, ginger, horseradish, licorice root, mustard.

The Digestive Herbs

Note: Many of the following descriptions include brewing instructions for tea. For convenience, measurements are given for one cup of tea, but in most cases you will want to multiply the ingredients by two to make a pint, or by four to make a quart. Double the amount of herb and extend brewing period for medicinal-strength tea.

AGRIMONY *(Agrimonis eupatoria).* This astringent, tonic, diuretic herb is a time-honored treatment for the liver, jaundice, diarrhea, fever, colds and asthma. Agrimony is especially healing to the mouth and throat. Maria Treben, the famous Austrian herbalist, wrote that gargling with agrimony tea clears the voice for singers and public speakers. Drink up to two cups daily for digestive problems, spleen disorders and as a liver tonic. Prepare the tea by infusion (pour 1 cup boiling water over 1 teaspoon tea; let stand 10 to 15 minutes).

ALLSPICE *(Pimento officinalis).* This sweet tropical spice, popular in cooking and baking, is an aromatic carminative and digestive stimulant. Used alone or in combination with other herbs, allspice eases flatulence and dyspeptic pain. Use it freely whenever a pleasant carminative is needed. To use in tea blends, crush or grind the seeds and do not boil for more than five minutes. This preserves the spice's volatile essential oils, which would otherwise escape during boiling. Combine 1 or 2 teaspoons crushed allspice in 1 cup water in a covered pan; bring just to a boil, simmer for 5 minutes or less, then remove from heat and let stand, covered, for 10 minutes before straining. Allspice can be added to any digestive blend. Use these same general instructions for the sweet spices cardamon *(Elattaria cardamomum)*, cinnamon *(Cinnamonomum zeylancium)* and cloves *(Eugenia caryophyllus).*

ALOE VERA. While the bitter sap of the rind of aloe vera contains cathartic principles, giving it dramatic laxative properties, the inner gel or juice of this healing plant is a digestive tonic that soothes internal organs. Aloe vera has been used in the treatment of ulcers, colitis and indigestion. Its popularity has produced several brands and product lines, including flavored aloe beverages. Whole-leaf products that are not filtered have a laxative effect; filtered whole-leaf juice and gel collected from the inner part of the leaf do not.

Studies at the Linus Pauling Institute of Science and Medicine show that six ounces of aloe vera juice taken three times daily increased protein digestion and absorption, decreased bowel putrefaction, improved pH levels in the intestinal tract and demonstrated antibacterial, antifungal and antiyeast activity.

Aloe vera's influence on stomach acidity has stimulated worldwide research on its usefulness in treating peptic ulcers.

ANGELICA *(Angelica archangelic)*. A popular European root used as a flavoring for candy, liqueurs (Benedictine and Chartreuse), Swedish bitters and the German product Underberg, angelica is an aromatic bitter. Its seeds are used to flavor wines, perfumes and vermouth. In addition to being an effective carminative (gas reliever), angelica has diuretic and antispasmodic effects; it is a well-documented treatment for dyspepsia, enteritis, flatulence and gastritis. Combine with chamomile to treat indigestion, flatulence and loss of appetite.

To brew angelica tea, make a decoction by simmering 1 teaspoon root per cup of water in a covered pot over low heat for 2 to 5 minutes after it reaches the boiling point, then let stand 15 minutes. If combining with chamomile or any herb that requires infusing, wait until the angelica decoction has simmered for 2 to 5 minutes, then remove cover, add the chamomile, replace the cover and let stand 15 minutes. This two-step procedure releases the medicinal ingredients in angelica root while preserving the more fragile volatile oils in chamomile blossoms.

Rosemary Gladstar warns that angelica tea is not recommended for pregnant women unless advised by a midwife or doctor.

ANISE *(Pimpinella anisum)*. Aniseed is an antispasmodic, carminative, anthelmintic and aromatic. Tea and tinctures containing it ease griping, intestinal colic and flatulence. Aniseed combines well with fennel and caraway for colic and flatulence. For tea, crush seeds just before using to release volatile oils. Pour 1 cup boiling water over 1 to 2 teaspoons seed, cover and let stand 5 to 10 minutes. The essential oil of aniseed can be taken internally by mixing 1 drop with a small amount of honey. Use as needed.

Follow these same instructions for similar aromatic, carminative seeds such as caraway seed (*Carum carvi*), celery seed (*Apium graveolens*), dill seed (*Antheium graveolens*) and fennel seed (*Foeniculum vulgare*).

ARROWROOT *(Maranta arundinacea).* Arrowroot, native to the Americas and West Indies, is a soothing demulcent and a nutritious food for children and invalids. Easy to swallow and pleasant in taste, the powdered rhizome contains over 80 percent starch. It is used as a thickening agent in cooking. American Indians used it to heal wounds from poisoned arrows, hence its name. Mix 1 or 2 tablespoons powdered root with juice or water to relieve nausea, vomiting or indigestion.

ARTICHOKE *(Cynar acolymus).* The familiar globe artichoke contains cynrin, recently isolated in research and shown to stimulate antitoxic liver functions. The key ingredient in Cynar aperitif, artichoke relieves dyspepsia and reduces blood fats. A tasty vegetable.

BLACK WALNUT HULL *(Juglans nigra).* Black walnut hull powders and tinctures are popular anthelmintics: They help expel worms and other parasites from the body. In addition, this astringent herb is an effective treatment for diarrhea. Walnut hulls are green when they fall from the tree in fall and turn black within a week. The green hulls of black walnut are prized for their superior benefits, making "green" black walnut hull tincture the preference of some herbalists.

BLESSED THISTLE *(Cnicus benedictus).* A "pure" (nonaromatic) bitter, blessed thistle has a long history of use as an appetite stimulant, digestive aid and liver tonic. It stimulates the secretion of bile and helps dispel flatulence. It is the key ingredient in the liqueur, Benedictine.

BURDOCK ROOT *(Arctium lappa).* An important herb for the liver, burdock root is a tonic, diuretic, demulcent herb. It is used to treat skin diseases, gout, kidney disease and bladder problems. Burdock root promotes kidney function and helps clear the blood of harmful acids. Research has shown that its seeds can lower blood sugar in rats, and in France, the fresh root is prescribed for this purpose.

Burdock root is a common Japanese vegetable called gobo, sold in thousands of grocery stores and sushi bars and used in many herbal formulas. Years ago a single batch of burdock was contaminated with belladonna root, which contains the poisonous compound atropine. It happened only once, but some medical authorities still refer to burdock as toxic because of its presumed atropine levels. Burdock root does not contain atropine, and it has a long and enviable track record of safe consumption by large numbers of people over long periods of time.

CALAMUS ROOT or SWEET FLAG *(Acorus calamus)*. An aromatic bitter, carminative, demulcent and antispasmodic, sweet flag or calamus root is widely used in Europe for indigestion, weakness of the digestive system, flatulence, colic, glandular disorders, dyspepsia, gastritis and gastric ulcers. The root, a rhizome, stimulates a sluggish stomach and intestine, dissipating excess mucus. It combines well with ginger and wild yam for colic and with meadowsweet and marshmallow for gastric conditions. The Austrian herbalist Maria Treben recommended making a cold infusion for calamus root tea. In addition, the dried root can be chewed to stimulate saliva, improve appetite and activate the entire digestive tract.

Calamus root was one of the herbs featured on the FDA's List of Unsafe Herbs, which was discontinued years ago because of its inaccuracies, and it is still listed in the U.S. Code of Federal Regulations as prohibited from direct addition to or use in human food. The controversy over calamus root stems from its asarone, a compound found to be carcinogenic in laboratory rats when taken in large quantities. Fritz Rudolf Weiss, M.D., a German authority on herbal medicine, wrote that calamus root has been popular from antiquity and is still widely used in Europe today without any reports of it causing cancer or any other problems. In *The New Age Herbalist,*

Richard Mabey wrote that rhizomes from Europe have low concentrations of asarone compared with those from India and no cases of malignancy have been reported in mill and mine workers who chew the rhizome daily. A conservative approach is to verify the source of calamus root and use this highly effective herb for short periods when needed.

CASCARA SAGRADA *(Rhamnus purshiana).* Cascara is a powerful laxative, a purgative if taken in sufficient doses and a bitter tonic. It is one of the oldest and most reliable remedies for chronic constipation. Cascara is not habit-forming but is a good intestinal tonic and remedy for gallstones and liver complaints. Caution: Do not use fresh bark; the dried bark should be at least one year old. To relieve constipation, make a tea by pouring 1 cup boiling water over 1 teaspoon bark and let it stand for one hour before drinking. Take on an empty stomach for best results.

CASTOR BEAN *(Ricinus communis),* CASTOR OIL PACKS. The castor bean, also called Palma Christi, is highly poisonous if swallowed and so is its oil unless extracted by carefully controlled cold pressing. The castor oil sold in pharmacies and health food stores is safe for internal use. Even though castor oil is still prescribed in small doses as a laxative, you won't find modern herbalists or holistic physicians making that recommendation.

It is the external use of cold-pressed castor oil that has made it a popular household remedy. Many apply it to warts, moles, liver spots, skin abrasions, external sores, ringworm, itching skin, hemorrhoids, abscesses and dandruff. Those are important applications, but it is the castor oil pack that has holistic healers most excited.

Castor oil packs were used in Eastern Europe during the 19th century for stomach disorders in adults and colic in babies. They were unknown in the United States until the American psychic, Edgar Cayce (1877-1945), recommended them for arthritis, colitis, intestinal impaction and other complaints.

Castor oil packs improve liver function, help normalize bowel function and enhance digestion.

To prepare a castor oil pack, start with a piece of wool flannel or a double thickness of cotton flannel about 18 inches square. A cloth diaper can be used for this purpose. Saturate the cloth with warmed castor oil, fold it to fit and apply it to the abdomen over the liver (above the navel) or, if desired, over the intestines (abdomen). Cover the pack with a sheet of plastic and place a heating pad or hot water bottle on top. If using a hot water bottle, cover everything with a towel for insulation. Leave the pack in place and keep it as hot as is comfortable for about an hour, then wipe off the excess oil and store the pack in a plastic bag. In most cases, daily treatment is recommended for one week, then intermittent treatment as desired.

CATNIP *(Nepeta cataria)*. A mild stimulant, antispasmodic, sedative, carminative and antacid, catnip has long been used to treat colic, flatulence, diarrhea and spasms. Catnip tea is safe for children and infants. Combining it with ginger root reinforces its stimulant properties; blending it with chamomile or lemon balm reinforces its sedative properties. For tea, brew an infusion of 1 cup boiling water poured over 1 teaspoon dried herb or 1 tablespoon fresh herb. Let stand 10 to 15 minutes.

CAYENNE PEPPER *(Capsicum annum)*. Hot peppers are a stimulant, tonic and pungent spice. They increase blood circulation, improve digestion, help relieve cramps and stop bleeding on contact. An important catalyst in herbal tea blending, cayenne pepper helps other herbs act faster. Because hot peppers burn the mouth, large doses can be placed in capsules and swallowed whole. To avoid a burning sensation in the stomach or esophagus, which may happen when you begin taking cayenne, swallow with food and follow with two large glasses of water.

CENTAURY *(Erythraea centaurium, Centaurium erythraea)*. This bitter gastric stimulant improves the appetite and strengthens the liver. Recommended for anorexia and dyspepsia, centaury improves circulation and has a tonic effect on the blood vessels.

CHAMOMILE *(Matricaria chamomilla)*. Also spelled camomile, chamomile is one of the most widely used herbs in the world. Even those who know little about its medicinal properties enjoy its fresh apple fragrance and relaxing influence. Chamomile is a carminative, tonic, sedative, antispasmodic, aromatic, stimulant and anthelmintic. According to Rudolf Weiss, M.D.:

> The medicinal value of chamomile is largely due to three actions: it reduces inflammation, relieves spasm and counteracts flatulence and the pain resulting from it. . . . The three actions make it clear why chamomile can have such a beneficial effect on acute stomach complaints. Relief is quite rapid, with pain reduced and the stomach and intestines settling down. Chamomile has also been found to encourage the healing of wounds. This effect is again closely linked with its anti-inflammatory action. Taking the two together, it is easy to see why chamomile is one of the best remedies for acute and chronic gastritis. The effect is not short-lived and purely symptomatic, but a genuine cure is achieved.

To brew chamomile tea for the treatment of indigestion or gas, be generous with your measurements. Use at least 2 to 3 teaspoons dried chamomile blossoms per cup of water. Do not boil the herb. Let stand, covered, 5 to 10 minutes before straining and serving. Drink 3 to 4 cups daily, preferably on an empty stomach before or between meals and again before retiring. For acute digestive discomfort or colic, sip hot chamomile tea slowly, drinking one cup every 20 to 30 minutes until symptoms subside.

A note on safety: According to Mark Blumenthal, executive director of the American Botanical Council, chamomile is frequently blamed for allergic reactions, especially in those who have severe ragweed allergies. But in the past 95 years, only five cases of chamomile allergy have been reported in the medical literature, and some research suggests that chamomile actually helps alleviate allergic reactions such as hay fever.

CHAPARRAL LEAF *(Larrea tridentata)*. This bitter herb from the Pacific Southwest is a diuretic, tonic, astringent, anti-inflammatory herb that protects against intestinal parasites and venomous bites. One of the best herbal antibiotics, chaparral leaf fights infections of the intestinal and urinary tracts, and it is effective in treating diarrhea caused by pathogens.

Because of actions by the U.S. Food and Drug Administration, chaparral has been labeled dangerous and pulled from many U.S. markets. On December 10, 1992, the agency issued a press release warning the public not to take chaparral because of its association with acute toxic hepatitis. Altogether, four people who took chaparral developed severe liver problems. In two cases, individuals consuming chaparral daily for several weeks suffered from jaundice and abdominal pain. In both cases, as well as in a third case documented by the Centers for Disease Control, the patients recovered after undergoing medical treatment and discontinuing their use of chaparral. In the fourth case, a patient with pre-existing liver damage took unknown quantities of chaparral and became gravely ill with liver and kidney failure.

The FDA concluded that chaparral "poses a potential health risk to the public, in particular to individuals with underlying liver damage due to acute or chronic disease." In response, health food stores stopped selling chaparral, and herbal tea makers removed it from their blends. Some tea blends were so popular that thousands of people were drinking them daily when the ban went into effect.

Did the FDA overreact? Considering that over 200 tons of chaparral were sold and presumably used by the general public between 1970 and 1990, and considering that at the time of the ban, chaparral was the primary ingredient in popular tea blends taken daily by thousands of Americans, four possible but unproven adverse reactions cannot be statistically significant.

In the two years that followed the chaparral scare, no additional cases of chaparral toxicity could be found. After an extensive review of chaparral's history, the Board of Trustees of the American Herbal Products Association voted in January 1995 to rescind its December 1992 recommendation that members voluntarily suspend the sale of chaparral. This decision was based on the findings of a panel of medical experts with specialties in gastroenterology and hepatitis and research from respected universities.

The American Herbal Products Association board recommends that member companies include the following notice when selling chaparral: "Seek advice from a health care practitioner before use if you have had, or may have had, liver disease. Discontinue use if nausea, fever, fatigue, or jaundice (e.g., dark urine, yellow discoloration of the eyes) should occur."

The next few years should see the gradual reintroduction of chaparral in health food stores and herbal tea catalogs. Most American herbalists support the conclusions of the American Herbal Products Association and welcome the return of this valuable plant.

Chaparral tea has a sharp, bitter creosote taste. It blends well with red clover and other herbs and should be infused for best results.

CHLORELLA *(green micro-algae).* A popular food supplement in Asia, this single-celled fresh-water algae from China is a source of high-grade protein, B-complex vitamins, enzymes and chlorophyll. Substantial research has documented health benefits including improved digestion, increased immune system function and improvement in chronic conditions. Chlorella tablets and powders can be an important source of concentrated nutrients for an impaired digestive system. Similar claims are made for spirulina, blue-green algae, powdered wheat grass juice and other dehydrated juice grasses.

CITRUS PEEL *(orange or tangerine peel).* Used in Chinese medicine as a stimulant, digestant, stomach tonic and to prevent nausea, citrus peel counteracts the formulation of mucus. It can be added to any herbal formula to improve digestion, relieve diarrhea or vomiting, treat indigestion and alleviate abdominal swelling. Citrus peel improves with drying and age, especially if peels are dried at low temperature and stored away from heat, light and humidity. Because citrus crops are usually treated with pesticides, purchase organically grown oranges or tangerines for this purpose. Add to decoctions after simmering and let stand for 5 to 10 minutes before serving; add to infusions before pouring boiling water over the plant material.

CLEAVERS *(Galium aparine)*. Also called bedstraw or galium, this common weed is a diuretic, tonic herb. Its tea has been used in the treatment of ulcers, urinary blockage, bladder infections and kidney stones. According to Maria Treben, bedstraw tea rids the liver, kidney, pancreas and spleen of toxic wastes. She recommended drinking it daily to tone the lymph glands and improve lymphatic disorders. Cleavers can be combined with other herbs and should be made as an infusion using fresh or dried plant material. Pour 1 cup boiling water over 1 teaspoon dried herb or 1 tablespoon fresh (double these measurements for medicinal strength tea) and let stand, covered, 10 to 15 minutes.

COMFREY *(Symphytum officinale)*. Every part of the comfrey plant is medicinal: its leaves, roots, stalks and flowers. A demulcent, astringent, nutritive, tonic, mucilaginous herb, comfrey has a soothing and healing effect on every organ it contacts. The only significant plant source of the cell-growth stimulator, allantoin, comfrey dramatically speeds the healing of wounds and even broken bones (hence its folk name, ''knit bone''). Among its hundreds of therapeutic applications are digestive disorders, urinary tract infections, diarrhea, hernias, hemorrhoids and ulcers.

Despite its long history and wide use, comfrey is widely reported to be toxic. How dangerous is it? Mark Blumenthal, executive director of the American Botanical Council and publisher of the journal *HerbalGram*, wrote:

> Recently the press created a scare about comfrey root. Comfrey contains a class of compounds that, when isolated and fed in large doses, can cause liver damage and cancer in rats. In hundreds of years of use, no cases of human problems with comfrey ever appeared. In 1984, however, there was a case of liver toxicity in a woman who had been taking comfrey-pepsin tablets. Soon after, warnings about comfrey began appearing in newspapers and magazines. The comfrey incident

might have looked different if it had been put into the context of a toxicity scale. One such scale is the HERP index, which classifies the cancer-causing potentials of various substances. Extrapolating from the HERP index, former U.S. Department of Agriculture botanist James Duke, Ph.D., calculated that less than one-fifth of an ounce of brown mustard is twice as cancer-causing as comfrey tea, which has roughly the same cancer-causing potential as a peanut butter sandwich. Wine is 144 times more cancer-causing than an equal amount of comfrey tea.

Canada was quick to ban comfrey sales, and FDA warnings removed comfrey tea from most health food stores in the U.S. Its final fate remains undecided. Comfrey continues to be an ingredient in herbal tea blends and it is sold by most herbal tea companies, though it may carry a warning label, "For external use only." Comfrey is so easy to grow and such a pleasant garden companion, you can insure an uninterrupted supply by planting your own.

Appreciating comfrey's long history of use and safety, However, in cases of liver disease, I would suggest alternative therapies, I can find no evidence suggesting that comfrey's risks outweigh its benefits in the treatment of gastritis, diverticulitis, irritable bowel syndrome, spastic colon, peptic or duodenal ulcers, leaky gut syndrome or Crohn's disease. In fact, many have found that its allantoin content, soothing mucilages and abundant nutrients make comfrey a "specific" for these disorders.

Though not widely known as a culinary herb, comfrey used to be a common ingredient in soups, stews, and salads. Dried comfrey root or leaves can be powdered and added to any juice or liquid to make a protein drink. Comfrey is said to be the second-highest vegetable source of protein; only the soy bean is a more concentrated source. It is also a source of soluble fiber.

Although most roots are decocted (brought to a boil, then simmered over low heat), comfrey is a fragile herb and should not be boiled. Instead, follow any of the following directions.

• *To make comfrey root tea:*

1. Make a cold infusion by soaking two teaspoons finely chopped root per cup of cold water overnight, or, to make a slow percolation infusion, place the chopped comfrey root in a muslin bag large enough to allow plenty of circulation, dampen the contents of the bag as you fill a glass jar with the water, then cap the jar, leaving the bag suspended at the top of the jar. Let stand overnight. Warm slightly in the morning and strain.

2. Make a hot water extract by combining 2 to 3 teaspoons chopped root per cup of cold water in a glass jar. Seal the jar and place it on a rack in a pot of hot water or in a crock pot partly filled with hot water and set on low temperature. Barely simmer the jar (water should not reach a rolling boil) for 2 to 4 hours before opening. Replenish evaporating water as needed.

• *To make comfrey leaf tea:* Pour boiling water over 1 heaping teaspoon dried leaf or 2 teaspoons fresh leaf per cup. Cover, let stand 10 to 15 minutes, and strain.

To add flavor to comfrey tea, add a small amount of peppermint leaf, rose hips, lemon balm, orange peel, spearmint, cinnamon, cloves, stevia or ginger. Comfrey combines well with other herbs and makes an important contribution to digestive blends.

• *To make comfrey mucilage,* an old remedy for lung ailments, digestive problems and internal hemorrhage,

Soak 2 ounces dried comfrey root in 1 quart of water overnight. Next morning, cover the pan, simmer over very low heat for 30 minutes (do not boil), then strain through cheesecloth or muslin. Add ¾ cup honey and ¼ cup vegetable glycerine, simmer 5 minutes, cool and store in a glass jar. Michael Tierra, author of *The Way of Herbs* recommends taking 2 tablespoons every hour for acute diseases, including internal hemorrhage; take 3 to 4 times daily for chronic ailments.

• *To make comfrey tincture,* fill a glass jar loosely with chopped fresh comfrey and add enough vodka or other 80-proof alcohol to cover the herb by 2 to 3 inches. Let stand in a warm place at least two weeks, shaking the jar daily. Strain and bottle. Store in a cool, dark place.

DANDELION *(Taraxacum officinale).* The familiar dandelion, from woody root to toothy leaf, is one of nature's most medicinal plants. Dandelion is a tonic herb for the digestive tract, a blood cleanser and a diuretic. Eat its fresh leaves in salads and drink dandelion tea for improved liver function. Michael Tierra notes that serious cases of hepatitis have been cured with the use of dandelion tea in combination with dietary restrictions in as little as one week.

Dandelion's bitter taste stimulates the production of bile. According to herbalist John Lust in *The Herb Book,* its fresh juice is most effective, but dandelion tea will also act as a liver tonic. To make dandelion leaf tea, steep 2 teaspoons dried leaves in 1 cup boiling water; let stand 10 minutes. To make dandelion root tea, combine 1 tablespoon chopped root with 1 cup water, bring to a boil, simmer over low heat in a covered pan for 10 to 15 minutes, remove from heat and let stand an additional 5 minutes. Drink before meals.

EPAZOTE *(Chenopodium ambrosiodes).* Also known as wormseed, this strongly scented herb is popular in Mexico and Guatemala as a seasoning for corn, black beans, fish and other foods. One small sprig supposedly renders beans "gas free," and the tea is used to relieve flatulence. Now naturalized in the southern U.S., epazote is sold in some markets as a seasoning for Mexican food.

FLAXSEED or LINSEED *(Linum usitatissiumum).* The crushed seeds of blue flowering flax are demulcent, mucilaginous, emollient and mildly laxative. They are used to treat inflamed mucous membranes, kidney irritation, gravel and painful urination. Flaxseeds can be ground and added to breads, cereals and other foods or sprouted and used as a salad ingredient. Flaxseed oil is a popular food supplement that adds essential fatty acids to the diet.

FO-TI *or* HO SHOU WU *(Polygonum multiflorum).* Fo-ti, a member of the buckwheat family, has an important place in

Chinese medicine, where it is considered an important herb for longevity. The plant can grow for over a hundred years and is said to improve with age. Its root is a liver tonic and diuretic; it strengthens the kidneys, liver and blood and plays an important role in the treatment of deficiency diseases, hypoglycemia and diabetes. Throughout China it is believed to prevent premature aging. Use the dried root to prepare a decoction: Simmer 2 teaspoons root in 1 cup water for 10 to 15 minutes in a covered pan. Drink before meals.

FRINGETREE *(Chionanthus virginicus).* The bark of the fringetree's root is a liver tonic, alterative, diuretic and laxative. It can be used safely for all liver problems, especially jaundice, and is considered a specific for gall bladder inflammation and gallstones. In the treatment of these disorders, fringetree root bark is often combined with barberry or wild yam. In *The Holistic Herbal,* David Hoffmann recommends brewing the tea as an infusion rather than a decoction. Pour 1 cup boiling water over 1 to 2 teaspoons bark; cover and let stand 10 to 15 minutes.

GENTIAN *(Gentiana lutes).* This "pure" bitter's flavor is so intense, it persists in dilutions of 1 part per 20,000. Its bitter glycosides make it Europe's most important bitter, and because it contains no tannin, it has no astringent or irritating effect. Gentian stimulates gastric secretions and acts as a tonic for the entire digestive tract, making heavy foods easier to digest; gentian-based bitters have been shown to be effective in curing indigestion and heartburn and stimulating the gallbladder and pancreas. Like most bitters, it is usually combined with other herbs. Gentian is an ingredient in most European bitters.

GERMANDER *(Teucrium chamaedrys).* This digestive tonic, antiseptic, diuretic, stimulant, astringent herb is effective in the treatment of fluid retention and digestive disorders. It is widely used in Arab countries in the treatment of ulcers and other gastrointestinal disturbances.

GINGER *(Zingiber officinale).* A "hot" bitter, this flavorful, knobby rhizome is enjoyed around the world in spicy main dishes, desserts, cookies and gingerbread. It's among the mostly widely used tea ingredients, both for its aromatic flavor and its warm, stimulating, carminative influence. Long prescribed in China for colds, flu, coughs, hangover, respiratory problems and kidney disease, ginger was more recently discovered in the West as a treatment for nausea. Both motion sickness and morning sickness respond to large doses of powdered ginger in capsules taken on an empty stomach. In addition, ginger has been shown to be effective in the treatment of ulcers and it increases circulation to the digestive organs. Safe for children, ginger is well-tolerated by almost everyone. Try adding dried ginger root to decoction blends and fresh, grated root to infusions.

GOLDENSEAL *(Hydrastis canadensis)*. A bitter, tonic, laxative, antiseptic and diuretic herb, goldenseal increases and improves the appetite by stimulating gastric secretions and the flow of bile. It is also a mild stimulant, toning and sustaining venous circulation. Goldenseal by itself or in blends is recommended for indigestion, stomach problems and liver disease. The American herbalist Jethro Kloss wrote that goldenseal has no superior when combined with myrrh, 4 parts goldenseal to 1 part myrrh, for an ulcerated stomach, duodenal ulcer or dyspepsia. Michael Tierra recommends taking goldenseal in capsules, two or three size 00 capsules daily for most conditions. Berberine, an ingredient in goldenseal, has been shown effective in the treatment of parasitic infections and diarrhea caused by bacteria.

GRAPEFRUIT SEED EXTRACT. An extract of grapefruit or other citrus seeds and the fruit's connecting membranes, this powerful antiseptic has been shown to kill bacteria, viruses, fungi, yeasts, parasites and other pathogens on contact. Sold in health food stores under the brand names ProSeed and Citricidal, grapefruit seed extract is available in very bitter-tasting drops or debittered powder capsules. Well-tolerated by people of all ages and having no known side effects when taken as recommended, grapefruit seed extract is effective in the treatment and prevention of traveler's diarrhea, infections of all types and chronic yeast infections.

HOPS *(Humulus lupulus).* The fruit or catkin of this flowering vine, best known as a beer ingredient and sleeping aid, is also a diuretic, stimulant, anthelmintic, alterative and astringent herb that promotes digestion by increasing the flow of bile. More commonly sold as a tincture than as a tea, hops helps lower blood sugar and has an antidiabetic effect.

HOREHOUND *(Marribium vulgare).* The leaves of this pleasant garden herb are sharply bitter. Best known as an old-fashioned cough drop ingredient, horehound is a tonic, bitter, slightly diuretic, aromatic, liver-tonic, stimulant, anthelmintic and culinary herb with a long history of use in the treatment of jaundice, worms, constipation, colic, stomachache, hepatitis and indigestion. Taken in large doses, it has a laxative effect.

HORSERADISH *(Amoracia rusticana).* A familiar culinary herb, horseradish is the root that brings tears to the eyes and clears the sinuses even without tasting it. Freshly cut or grated horseradish and, to a lesser extent, commercially prepared horseradish, stimulates the flow of bile and activates the gall bladder and liver. Take the fresh root only in small quantities as it's a powerful stimulant and can cause disorienting nausea. Horseradish root is a stimulant, mild laxative and diuretic. It improves digestion and helps ease flatulence and stomach cramps. Wasabi, a green Japanese horseradish, is the spice that makes sushi an eye-watering experience. Wasabi powder, sold in health food stores and Oriental markets, is mixed with water to form a pungent green paste for condiment use, and a pinch added to any herbal tea acts as a catalyst and tonic.

ICELAND MOSS *(Centaria islandica).* A lichen, Iceland moss is a traditional remedy for coughs and chronic stomach complaints. Often confused with Irish moss, Iceland moss contains bitter ingredients that activate the liver. As John Lust reported, this plant must be boiled for long periods to release its nutrients and, if used in excessive doses or for prolonged periods, it can cause gastrointestinal irritation and liver problems.

IRISH MOSS *(Chondrus crispus)*. A widely used seaweed, Irish moss is a source of water-soluble fiber that reduces irritation in the intestines, reduces sensitivity to gastric acid and relaxes painful urinary spasms. Demulcent, emollient and nutritive, Irish moss can be combined with licorice, lemon, cinnamon or other flavors. To brew the decoction, soak 1 tablespoon moss in cold water for 15 minutes to soften, then simmer in 3 cups water for 10 to 15 minutes, covered, over low heat. Let stand another 5 minutes before straining.

JUNIPER BERRIES *(Juniperus communis)*. These fragrant, pleasant-tasting berries, best known as an ingredient in gin, are diuretic, aromatic, stimulant, carminative, antiseptic and a tonic for the stomach. If you gather them yourself, collect the dark, older berries that have dried on the bush for best results. Juniper berries increase the appetite, aid digestion and, their major use, increase urination. Rudolf Weiss, the German physician, wrote that juniper irritates the kidneys and should never be taken for more than six weeks without interruption. The legendary Father Kneipp, a 19th-century German physician and priest, used 1 or 2 berries a day in tea on the first day of therapy, building up to 15 berries on the tenth day, then back down to 2 per day on the twentieth. "This really cleanses the kidneys," wrote Bernard Jensen in *Nature Has a Remedy* "and is good for the liver, blood cleansing, weak stomach, foul breath, gas, urethral infection, bladder stones and as a stimulant." Brew the tea as an infusion, combining juniper berries with other herbs as desired. The berries can also be chewed or added to food.

KUDZU or KUZU *(Pueraria pseudohirsuta)*. Called *pueraria* or *ko ken* in Chinese medicine, the kudzu is best known in the U.S. as an obnoxious vine that now covers the South, where it was planted as an experimental cattle food. Whole kudzu root recently made headlines by reducing alcoholic cravings in laboratory animals. It is valuable as a digestive aid because of its antispasmodic, demulcent properties. It neutralizes stomach acid and helps relieve gastrointestinal distress. Whole kudzu root is available from herbalists for use as a decoction (simmer the root 10 to 15 minutes over low heat in a covered pan) and can be combined with ginger, licorice, cinnamon or other herbs for best results. The refined kudzu starch sold in health food stores is imported from Japan, where it is a popular thickening agent similar to cornstarch.

LAVENDER *(Lavendula* varieties). Lavender is not highly regarded as a digestive aid in its own right, but it can be a valuable supportive ingredient in blends. The blossoms are aromatic and relaxing. Brew as an infusion.

LEMON BALM *(Melissa officinalis).* This pleasant-tasting member of the mint family is an antispasmodic, sedative, carminative and aromatic therapy for indigestion, stomach cramps and flatulence. Use alone or in combination with chamomile, ginger, peppermint and other herbs. According to Rudolf Weiss, small doses are most powerful for relieving spasms and nervous tension; increasing the dosage does not increase its effect. Brew as an infusion. Safe for all ages.

LICORICE ROOT *(Glycyrrhiza glabra).* Most familiar as an ingredient in black candy ropes and other confections, licorice root is so sweet and aromatic that it's often used to flavor herbal teas. Because of its relaxing effect on the digestive tract, especially the stomach, it is an effective treatment for ulcers. It is also recommended for the symptoms of adrenal exhaustion, stress, hypoglycemia and chronic fatigue.

Unfortunately, licorice has side effects. Glycyrrhizin, its most active principle, can cause edema (fluid retention), heartburn, and, in some people, headaches. These side effects are well-documented in German medical texts, for licorice has long been prescribed by that country's physicians for ulcers and stomach pain. One common side effect of licorice overconsumption is a round "moon face" caused by fluid retention. In Europe, licorice roots are now treated to remove their glycyrrhizin content, but in the

U.S. and Canada, the roots are sold untreated. You can, however, purchase deglycyrrhinized licorice capsules, tinctures and other preparations in health food stores. Because of its effectiveness, deglycyrrhinized licorice is beginning to appear in over-the-counter products for the treatment of heartburn and acid indigestion.

To use licorice for therapeutic purposes, such as the treatment of ulcers or to prevent anxiety and stress, it is better to take deglycyrrhizined licorice than to drink large quantities of strongly brewed tea. A daily cup of beverage-strength licorice root tea isn't likely to cause problems, but several cups per day could do so in sensitive people. In small doses and for occasional use, adverse side effects are unlikely.

MALLOW *(Malva vulgaris).* Mallow tea is used in Europe for inflammations of the mucous membranes, bladder problems, gastrointestinal irritations, gastritis and ulcers. Its demulcent, anti-inflammatory, astringent properties make it similar to marshmallow, which is usually considered a stronger, more effective herb. However, mallow can be a valuable ingredient in blends for improved digestion. Brew mallow leaves and flowers as an infusion and the root as a decoction.

MARSHMALLOW *(Althea officinalis).* Marshmallow root is a demulcent, emollient, mucilaginous herb and one of the best sources of easily digested vegetable mucilage. High in pectin, a soluble fiber, marshmallow root soothes inflamed or irritated intestines. Brew as a decoction.

MEADOWSWEET *(Filipendula ulmaria).* A stomach tonic, antacid, anti-inflammatory, and astringent, meadowsweet is one of the best digestive remedies available. It reduces stomach acidity, relieves nausea and heartburn, treats peptic ulcers and relieves diarrhea in children. As the British herbalist David Hoffmann observed, meadowsweet contains an aspirinlike chemical that calms inflammation as well as another ingredient that soothes intestinal lining, making this a pleasant alternative to aspirin, which can cause bleeding and ulcers. In addition, it increases the intestinal lining's ability to absorb nutrients.

MILK THISTLE *(Carduus marianus).* Milk thistle seed preparations are best sellers in health food stores because they are such effective liver stimulants, tonics and healers. This is one herb that truly reverses liver damage. Important in the treatment of mushroom poisoning, hepatitis, alcoholic cirrhosis, drug damage and the damage caused by environmental toxins, milk thistle has been scientifically researched in Europe for over 45 years. In addition to improving the liver, milk thistle seed can be used for all gall bladder problems. Brew the seeds as an infusion, grind them and add them to food, or take milk thistle seed capsules or tinctures.

MYRRH *(Commiphora myrrha).* A plant resin best known as a biblical incense, myrrh is an antiseptic, astringent, carminative and stomach tonic. Bitter in taste, it is often combined with goldenseal for colds and flu. Myrrh contains aromatic volatile oils that relieve flatulence and stimulate digestion. Most health food stores carry myrrh tincture, and myrrh resin can be ordered from herbal supply shops, aromatherapy companies and incense sellers. Add to infusions or add a dropperful of tincture to tea after brewing.

OATS *(Avena sativa).* Oat straw and oats are a wonderful nutritive tonic for the nervous system; oat straw tea helps calm frazzled nerves, and all oat preparations (oatmeal, oat muffins, etc.) contain soluble fibers that enhance digestion. The slippery white mucilage that appears when you cook oatmeal is oat gum, a gentle emollient for the entire digestive tract. Oat straw tea should be made as an infusion; it combines well with chamomile, lemon balm and other relaxing herbs.

OREGON GRAPE ROOT *(Berberia aquifolium).* A mild stimulant, liver tonic, laxative, diuretic and nerve tonic, Oregon grape root is one of the best blood purifiers and liver stimulants. It helps relieve constipation and has mild antiseptic properties. Oregon grape root is not recommended during pregnancy. Brew as a decoction: simmer 1 or 2 teaspoons root in 1 cup water for 10 to 15 minutes over low heat, tightly covered. Remove from heat and let stand another 5 minutes.

PAPAYA *(Carica papaya)*. This familiar tropical fruit contains a protein digesting enzyme known as papain, which resembles the animal enzyme pepsin. Papain is used as a meat tenderizer. Bernard Jensen recommended making a tea from dried papaya seeds (simmer 1 tablespoon dry seeds in 1 cup water for a minute or two) as a digestive tonic.

PEPPERMINT *(Mentha piperita)*. An aromatic herb, peppermint contains volatile essential oils that improve digestion, alleviate flatulence and relieve feelings of fullness by speeding the transit of food through the stomach.

David Hoffmann recommends only one herb for the treatment of Crohn's disease, and that is peppermint, an opinion seconded by David Williams, M.D., in the March 1995 issue of his *Alternatives* newsletter. "Peppermint leaves and oil," wrote Williams, "were probably put on this earth specifically to treat gastrointestinal disorders." In Europe, peppermint is widely used for stomach, liver, gallbladder and pancreatic disturbances. It should be taken only when needed; Williams warns that regular, habitual use lessens its effect. He added:

> Most physicians and herbalists don't realize that the active menthol ingredients in peppermint are rapidly absorbed in the stomach and upper gastrointestinal tract. Taking peppermint in the form of tea, oil or tincture will have little, if any, effect on the lower bowels. With problems like IBS, enteric-coated peppermint oil capsules must be used to deliver the active ingredients to the colon. European studies have found that enteric-coated capsules are very effective in treating the disease. Doctors in this country who scoff at the use of peppermint for treating IBS are undoubtedly unfamiliar with the European use of enteric-coated products. The dosage generally recommended for IBS patients has been two to three capsules

a day taken between meals. The only side effect noted has been a temporary burning sensation in the rectal area after a bowel movement. This comes from excess unabsorbed menthol. It poses no danger and can be alleviated by simply reducing the dosage.

QUASSIA *(Picrasma excelsor)*. These wood chips are a bitter tonic that is an excellent remedy for indigestion. It increases the appetite and has been used with some success in the treatment of anorexia nervosa. Quassia's primary use is as an anthelmintic: It expels threadworms when taken as a tea or enema. David Hoffmann recommends brewing the tea by cold infusion, soaking 1 tablespoon of wood chips in 1 cup water overnight.

RHUBARB ROOT *(Rheum palmatum)*. Also called Turkey rhubarb root, this plant is *not* the familiar red-stalked garden vegetable. A bitter stomach tonic, mild purgative and astringent, it has a cleansing action on the entire digestive tract and speeds elimination. Rhubarb root may color the urine red or yellow. David Hoffmann recommends combining it with carminative herbs such as chamomile, peppermint or ginger. Brew as a decoction, simmering ½ to 1 teaspoon root in 1 cup water for 10 to 15 minutes; let stand another 5 minutes before serving.

SARSAPARILLA *(Similax officinalis)*. Sarsaparilla's familiar root beer taste makes it a pleasant addition to herbal tea blends, and its diuretic, tonic, stimulant, demulcent and carminative properties make it an important digestive tonic. Jethro Kloss considered it an excellent antidote for poisons and found it useful in treating rheumatism, skin eruptions and ringworm. He recommended taking the tea (1 to 2 cups daily) or tincture (25 to 50 drops daily) for no more than two weeks out of every three. Michael Tierra advised combining sarsaparilla with sassafras and yellow dock as a spring tonic. According to him, a hot decoction (2 tablespoons root boiled in 2 cups water) acts as a powerful agent to expel gas from the stomach and intestines.

SASSAFRAS ROOT BARK *(Sassafras officinale)*. An aromatic, diuretic and stimulant, sassafras is a blood purifier and is used in the treatment of skin diseases, ulcers, diarrhea and kidney problems. Often called a spring tonic herb, it cleanses the entire system. Its aromatic oils provide a flavor that improves many herbal blends, and these same oils relieve gas and colic. Taken warm, sassafras tea relieves spasms.

Sassafras contains safrole, a substance that the FDA tested in large quantities on rats in the 1950s. When the rats developed liver cancer, sassafras was blamed. The same compound, safrole, is found in nutmeg, black pepper, and mace, but these seasonings were never implicated. Because safrole is not soluble in water, someone drinking sassafras tea will ingest very little of it, and no case of liver damage from sassafras tea has ever been reported. In fact, the southeastern U.S., where most sassafras tea is consumed, has a lower liver cancer rate than other parts of the country.

SAVORY *(Satureia hortensis)*. Also called summer savory, this warming, aromatic herb was once considered the best possible remedy for colic and flatulence. In cooking, it has a special affinity for beans. Use in foods, blend with other teas, or prepare an infusion of the leaves.

SENNA *(Cassia marilandica)*. Also called American senna or the locust plant, senna is a valuable laxative. It is recommended for indigestion, bad breath, a bad taste in the mouth and in the treatment of intestinal parasites. Because senna by itself can cause cramps or spasms, it should be combined with aromatic, carminative herbs such as chamomile and ginger. As an anthelmintic it works best in combination with other herbs in that category. To brew a decoction,

> Bring 4 tablespoons senna to a boil with 2 cups water and 1 teaspoon powdered ginger, 1 tablespoon fresh grated ginger and/or 1 teaspoon fennel seed. Simmer over low heat, tightly covered, for 30 minutes; then remove from heat and let stand another 10 minutes. Drink 2 ounces (⅛ cup) at a time.

Take this herb in small doses as it is a more powerful laxative than cascara sagrada. In most cases, it relieves constipation within six to eight hours. Senna is not recommended for use during pregnancy or by the elderly.

SLIPPERY ELM BARK *(Ulmus fulva).* The inner bark of the slippery elm tree is a demulcent, emollient, nutritive, diuretic, slightly astringent and tonic source of mucilaginous, water-soluble fiber. It can be prepared like oatmeal to nourish the body while relieving stomach complaints. A small amount of powdered bark in water forms a thick jelly, similar to psyllium husk powder.

SPEARMINT *(Mentha spicata* or *M. aquatica).* Thanks to the popularity of spearmint chewing gums, breath mints, toothpastes and mouthwashes, spearmint is as well-known as its cousin, peppermint. Both are digestive aids that help prevent flatulence. Spearmint is also a mild diuretic that helps alleviate fluid retention.

STEVIA *(Stevia rebaudiana).* Although it has nothing to do with improving digestion, stevia has much to do with improving the taste of herbal teas. Stevia is widely used in Europe, South America and Asia as a sugar substitute, but the U.S. Food and Drug Administration does not allow it to be labeled as a sweetener; in fact, for a while the FDA banned the herb's importation. The stevia ban has been lifted, and this herb is likely to attract a wider audience in years ahead. In a typical blend of herbal tea, stevia might account for 1 percent of the total. Use just a pinch when experimenting. Stevia contains no sugar, has no documented adverse side effects and is safe for diabetics.

STONE ROOT *(Collinsonia canadensis).* Stone root is a diuretic and antilithic; as its name suggests, it is mainly used in the treatment and prevention of urinary gravel, kidney stones and gallstones. A strong diuretic, it is often combined with parsley or other antilithic herbs to encourage the passing of stones or gravel. Brew as a decoction.

VIOLET *(Viola odorata).* The entire plant is mucilaginous, laxative, alterative and antiseptic. Violet leaf tea is a healing blood purifier and gives prompt relief to internal ulcers. Jethro Kloss wrote that violet combines well with red clover, another blood purifier. Violet is of interest to researchers because it relieves pain much like aspirin, but without aspirin's side effects. This is a soothing herb for the digestive system. Brew as an infusion.

WAHOO ROOT BARK *(Eunoymus atropurpureus).* The bark of the wahoo root is a circulatory stimulant, diuretic, laxative and liver tonic. It removes congestion from the liver and stimulates the free flow of bile; in addition, it is useful in the treatment of jaundice, gall bladder disease, gallstones and constipation.

WOOD BETONY *(Betonica officinalis).* This aromatic, carminative, astringent herb is an effective and relaxing stomach tonic. A strong decoction kills intestinal parasites, relieves intestinal gas, treats bladder and kidney problems and alleviates back pain and stitches in the side. Wood betony is sometimes used as a substitute for black tea, with which it shares a similar flavor, but the herb lacks black tea's caffeine and acidity. To brew a medicinal decoction, bring 2 tablespoons herb to a boil in 2 cups water; cover and simmer over low heat for 5 minutes. For a beverage infusion, pour 2 cups boiling water over 1 tablespoon herb, cover and let stand 10 minutes.

WORMWOOD *(Artemisia absinthium).* An important bitter herb, wormwood lives up to its name by helping rid the body of intestinal parasites. In addition, its antiseptic, antispasmodic, carminative and stimulant properties make it a tonic for the stomach and digestive tract. The essential oil of wormwood is toxic and addictive, which is how Absinthe, the notorious liqueur, ruined some of the best minds in Europe a hundred years ago. Wormwood tea and powdered wormwood capsules are considered safe in small quantities even for prolonged use; in more concentrated doses, such as in the treatment of intestinal worms, it can be taken for several days.

YELLOW DOCK ROOT *(Rumex crispus)*. The root of this nuisance weed is a buried treasure, one of the best-known blood purifiers in herbal medicine. A gentle laxative, yellow dock root stimulates bile production and helps tone the liver. Like burdock root and dandelion root, yellow dock root improves digestion and the assimilation of nutrients, stimulates the elimination of toxins from the body and gradually restores normal body function.

STRATEGIES FOR IMPROVED DIGESTION

Beneficial Bitters

Bitters are exactly what they sound like: bitter tasting herbs. Humans have used them for thousands of years to improve digestion and stimulate the appetite. You'll find them mentioned in the Bible and in the medical records of every civilization, ancient and modern.

Our tongues can detect four kinds of taste: sweet, sour, bitter and salty. In modern America, our sweet and salty taste buds see most of the action, for we are culturally conditioned to avoid sour and bitter tastes. In Europe and other parts of the world, bitters are alive and well, and all of us would benefit from a greater exposure to these sharp, pungent flavors. As soon as taste buds detect something bitter, they stimulate the secretion of gastric juices, such as bile from the liver. In addition, they have a tonic action on the entire body.

Bitters that improve digestion can be classified into three categories: tonic, aromatic and hot. Tonic bitters, like gentian root and blessed thistle, are the sharpest tasting and have an immediate effect on the digestive process. Aromatic bitters, like angelica root, myrrh gum and peppermint, are more fragrant and contain volatile oils. Hot bitters, like ginger root and horseradish, stimulate circulation in the stomach, intestines, sinuses and throughout the body.

Bitters are essential ingredients in Campari, Cynar, Magnoberta Fernet and other European aperitifs. A small amount taken before and after eating is a time-honored means of improving digestion.

Most Americans have heard of Angostura bitters, a widely sold aromatic preparation of water, alcohol, gentian and harmless vegetable flavorings, extractives and vegetable coloring matter, as its label says. Named not for the angostura tree or its bark but rather for Angostura, Venezuela, the town in which it was invented in 1830, Angostura bitters can be used as a sodium-free food seasoning, cocktail ingredient or appetite stimulant, and it can be taken after dinner to improve digestion and prevent flatulence.

Angostura is our best-selling digestive bitter because it really isn't bitter at all. Compared to European bitters, the Angostura blend is sweet and mild. Bitters are an acquired taste, to say the least. For a jolting taste sensation, try a tablespoon of Swedish bitters—and not the mild form sold in American health food stores, but the stronger, more effective version you can make yourself.

The late Austrian herbalist Maria Treben made Swedish bitters a household name in Europe after she discovered its recipe in an old manuscript, which appears in her book *Health Through God's Pharmacy*, as follows.

Swedish Bitters Recipe Combine 10 grams aloe (or substitute gentian root or wormwood powder), 5 grams myrrh, 0.2 grams saffron, 10 grams senna leaves, 10 grams natural camphor, 10 grams rhubarb root, 10 grams zedoary root, 10 grams manna, 5 grams carline thistle root, 10 grams angelica root, and 10 grams Theriac venezian. Place this mixture in a wide-mouth two-quart bottle and add 1.5 quarts of 80-proof or higher proof alcohol (vodka, brandy, rum, whatever you prefer). Seal the jar and let it stand in the sun or near a stove or other warm place for at least 14 days (longer is better), shaking the jar daily. Strain the liquid, pour into small bottles and store in a cool, dark place.

As Maria Treben wrote, "This way it can be kept for many years. The longer it stands, the more effective it becomes. Shake well before use!"

The resulting product has far too many uses to list here, ranging from the treatment of stomach cramps and indigestion to external application as a poultice or for insect bites or mouth sores. It's no exaggeration to say that Treben found a hundred effective uses for this tincture, which she credited with saving her life. Though not the worst tasting liquid you'll ever encounter, Swedish bitters does live up to its name and it's an acquired taste: strong, pungent, and yes, very bitter.

It is difficult if not impossible to obtain the ingredients in Treben's Swedish Litters in the U.S. Fortunately, you can order them directly from the Austrian company licensed by Maria Treben to manufacture the blend, and its quality is unsurpassed.

To order, send $20 in U.S. funds to RiPharm, P. O. Box 23, 4710 Grieskirchen, Austria, or write first to verify price and availability. As this product is not distributed in the U.S. or England, there is no English-language labeling. I add 1-¼ quarts (5 cups) of 80-proof vodka to the contents of one box. Any distilled liquor of at least 80-proof will work well; you can substitute rum, brandy or other alcohols as desired. Seal the jar tightly and leave it in a warm place, shaking it daily. Maria Treben's instructions recommend letting the jar stand for 14 days, but the blend's flavor and intensity increase substantially if you leave it for four weeks or longer. To use, strain the tincture through cheesecloth and store it in tightly closed amber glass bottles away from heat and light. Properly stored, the tincture will keep indefinitely.

To use Swedish bitters for improved digestion, take 1 teaspoon diluted with water or straight from the spoon in the morning and evening, shortly before breakfast and dinner. For best results, hold the bitters on your tongue for half a minute or more before swallowing. It takes getting used to, but the benefits are often dramatic. For indigestion after eating, take up to 3 tablespoons straight or diluted with water, as needed. For serious ailments, dilute 1 tablespoon in ½ cup herb tea and take half of this before eating and the other half after, repeating the treatment with every meal.

If you'd like to explore European aperitifs, they are easy to find, especially in liquor stores that carry a large inventory. One Italian product that resembles Maria Treben's is Magnoberta Fernet, which contains aloe, quinine, gentian, rhubarb, zedoary, myrrh, chamomile, licorice, cardamon, galangal, centaury, imperatoria, angelica, calumba, saffron, and peppermint oil.

The Fiber Factor

Dietary fiber, what remains of indigestible plant cell walls after food moves through the small intestine, is important because it makes stools soft and bulky, speeding their transit time through the large intestine. This dilutes the effects of any toxic or carcinogenic compounds in the intestine, causing them to be excreted quickly, and it helps remove or inhibit toxic bacteria in the colon. Good colon health depends on fiber. The lack of it has been linked to constipation, diverticulitis, diabetes, gastrointestinal disorders, heart disease, colon cancer and obesity.

Soluble fibers dissolve in water; insoluble or crude fibers do not. Both are necessary for optimum digestion. In fact, there are five types of fiber—cellulose, hemicellulose, pectin, gums and lignin—all of which enhance digestion and elimination. Soluble fibers such as oat bran absorb cholesterol and toxins, while insoluble fibers add bulk, speeding the transit of fecal matter through the colon. Low-fiber diets are the leading cause of diverticulitis, irritable bowel syndrome, constipation, colon cancer and hemorrhoids.

Sources of soluble fiber include whole fresh and dried fruit, dried peas, lentils, beans, barley, oats, guar gum, pectin, oat gum and psyllium husks. Psyllium is the active ingredient in Metamucil, the popular fiber laxative. Wheat bran is an insoluble fiber, and so is the roughage found in many vegetables and other whole grains. When you increase the fiber content of your diet, do it gradually and increase your consumption of water at the same time. If you don't, or if you overwhelm a weak digestive system with too much fiber, the result can be intestinal blockage. Gradually replace white flour bread and pasta with whole grain products, eat whole fruits and vegetables and replace white rice with brown or blend the two together.

Those who suffer from diverticulitis, Crohn's disease, irritable bowel syndrome, spastic colon and similar ailments must approach fiber with caution. In advanced cases, even the gentlest soluble fibers can cause problems. Although fiber is an important part of the cure for these illnesses, a depleted and damaged digestive tract must be healed before it can cope with whole foods. Fresh, raw juices are probably the best initial therapy for these patients.

A note on psyllium: This popular, effective bulking agent is a potential allergen. Some nurses who prepare daily doses in hospitals or nursing homes have inhaled enough of the powder to develop serious allergies. Psyllium comes from *Plantago ovata,* a member of the plantain family (plantain the garden weed, not the tropical green banana) and, as with any plant, too much of it can cause an adverse reaction. When measuring psyllium husk powder, keep your face averted or wear a pollen mask. Add a teaspoon or tablespoon of powder to a full glass of juice or water, stir briskly and swallow the liquid before it gels. Follow with another glass of water. Some commercial psyllium powders contain acidophilus bacteria to protect intestinal flora. If you use plain psyllium powder, recommended because it does not contain the sugar and artificial flavors found in Metamucil and similar brands, take an acidophilus supplement at the same time.

Fiber supplements that can be taken in capsules or used like powdered psyllium husk include glucomannan (*Amorphophallus konjac* and *A. riveri*), a powdered root that absorbs up to 40 times its weight in liquids, giving a feeling of fullness that aids dieters and improves bowel function; guar gum (*Cyamopsis tetragonolaba*), a thickening agent from the seeds of the Indian Cluster Bean or Guar plant with similar properties; and pectin, the familiar jelling agent used in jams and jellies. Agar agar, a seaweed, is another source of soluble fiber, but it requires cooking for best results. Agar agar is popular as a mineral-rich vegetarian substitute for Jell-O. All are available through health food stores.

Eliminate Parasites

Roundworms, threadworms, tapeworms, flukes and flatworms are some of the animals that seek a comfortable home in human beings. They come in all sizes, from large intestinal worms to the tiny *Giardia lamblia* that infests most of the lakes and ponds of North America and cryptosporidium, which caused 400,000 people to become ill when it contaminated Milwaukee's water supply in Wisconsin. The Environmental Protection Agency considers cryptosporidium the leading cause of waterborne illness in the U.S., with problems reported across the country. Both *Giardia* and cryptosporidium cause severe flu-like symptoms.

Parasites are a special concern in kindergartens and day-care centers, where fecal contamination can spread quickly. They are the bane of travelers (unfamiliar microbes in foreign countries often cause diarrhea) and of hikers or campers who stay closer to home (*Giardia* again). Refugees and immigrants from parasite-ridden areas sometimes carry micro-organisms without having symptoms themselves; when they work in restaurants, private homes, nursing homes or day-care centers, they may unknowingly spread parasites to others. Raw seafood, undercooked pork and exotic foods prepared raw pose parasite risks. So do household pets. Even antibiotics have been blamed for our parasite problems because they kill beneficial bacteria that help repel parasites from healthy bodies. In the stomach, low levels of hydrochloric acid (HCl) allow some parasites to survive.

The symptoms of parasite infestation range from dramatic bouts of diarrhea, vomiting, cramping and other flu-like symptoms to conditions so minor they go unnoticed or are mistaken for mild indigestion. Anyone who suffers from digestive problems, and even those who don't, may want to ensure that they aren't playing host to intestinal worms or other parasites.

Obviously, severe symptoms require medical attention. But if you experience adverse side effects from prescription drugs that kill parasites, or if you have mild symptoms or simply want to be sure you aren't providing a cozy home for parasites, the following strategy is likely to be effective.

Seven Day Cure

First, spend a few days eating foods that worms don't like, such as onions, garlic, pickles, pumpkin seeds, sage, fennel, thyme, cloves and salt; while avoiding the foods they thrive on, which are sugar, carbohydrates, dairy products and grains containing gluten (wheat, rye, oats and barley). Ann Louise Gittelman, author of *Guess What Came to Dinner: Parasites and Your Health* recommends that you:

- Avoid raw fruits and vegetables (drink their juice or cook them during the week of treatment)
- Avoid cold or iced foods and drinks because these all cause the intestines to contract
- Take two or more HCl tablets or capsules with each meal if you have an insufficiency of this essential digestive fluid (which she considers likely if you are over age 40, have type A blood or are a strict vegetarian)
- Take digestive enzymes such as bromelains, papain and protease with every meal. In addition, support your system with blood-cleansing herbs such as red clover, chaparral, yellow dock, dandelion root or burdock root, all of which help rid the blood and lymph of toxins generated by parasites. Take these herbs in teas, tinctures or capsules.

In *Natural Healing with Herbs* Humbart Santillo recommended taking 2 chaparral tablets every 4 hours for one day, then 1 tablet every 4 hours for one week for this purpose.

After three to five days of preparation, continue taking chaparral and, in addition, take 2 wormwood capsules 3 times daily for three days, or substitute another anthelmintic herb. In addition, take 2 or 3 dry grapefruit seed extract capsules three times daily or fill empty gelatin capsules with liquid grapefruit seed extract just before swallowing. Grapefruit seed extract may be the safest, most effective anthelmintic available. Continue to eat extra garlic or take several garlic capsules during the day. Quassia chips, the white rind and seeds of pomegranate and black walnut hull tincture are effective anthelmintics and can be used in place of wormwood. All of the deworming herbs mentioned here are safe to take in tea or capsules for short periods. If any anthelmintic herb disagrees with you, substitute something that doesn't.

On the fourth day of herbal therapy, drink a cup of senna tea, which has a laxative effect; add licorice root or chamomile to the tea to prevent cramping. In addition, take extra fiber to "scrub" the intestines clean.

This one-week therapy is likely to dislodge most intestinal parasites and leave you feeling much improved. For another herbal parasite therapy which is popular in the U.S. and Canada, see *The Cure for All Cancers* by Hulda Clark, Ph.D. Dr. Clark's treatment combines wormwood, cloves and black walnut hull tincture made from fresh green hulls and is effective, she claims, for every type of internal parasite.

To be sure you are free of parasites, you can arrange for testing through the Great Smokies Diagnostic Laboratory in Asheville, N.C. (phone 1-800-522-4762). This lab specializes in parasitology testing and can provide referrals to health care practitioners in your area.

To prevent future infestations, follow these commonsense steps. Wash your hands carefully, especially under fingernails, after changing diapers, handling raw meat or playing with pets. Do what you can to prevent worms and other parasites in your dogs and cats. I give my Lab, Samantha, grapefruit seed extract capsules every day because she swims in a *Giardia* infested lake; her frequent stool samples, tested because of her work as a therapy dog in hospitals and nursing homes, show her to be free of all parasites.

Disinfect raw fruits, vegetables, meats and eggs by soaking them for several minutes in a sink full of cold water plus several drops of grapefruit seed extract, a tablespoon of food-grade hydrogen peroxide or original formula Clorox bleach (use ½ teaspoon per gallon of water), then rinse in plain water.

Take grapefruit seed capsules daily and while traveling use liquid grapefruit seed extract to disinfect drinking water. A drop or two in a glass of water kills all viruses, bacteria, yeasts, molds, fungi, parasites and microbes within a few seconds. The taste may be bitter, but it is very reassuring.

Supplement your diet with hydrochloric acid, digestive enzymes and garlic. Avoid sugar and sweet fruits (pineapple, cranberries and papaya are exempt as they contain antiparasitic enzymes), avoid refined carbohydrates, eat high-fiber foods and take acidophilus and similar supplements to increase your supply of beneficial bacteria.

Finally correct any nutritional deficiencies or imbalances with appropriate supplements, such as vitamins, minerals, trace elements and enzymes. A healthy body and strong immune system are your best defense against parasites.

TUMMY TROUBLE: THE DIRTY DOZEN

COLIC

Colic—spasmodic abdominal pains in young infants and children accompanied by irritability or crying—also refers to conditions of flatulence and other symptoms of indigestion in infants up to three months in age. Its causes include overfeeding, swallowing air or emotional upset, but its primary cause is probably dietary. According to pediatrician Lendon Smith, cow's milk formulas such as SMA, Similac and Enfamil may precipitate colic, diarrhea, rashes, ear infections, asthma and other conditions in up to 50 percent of infants. Breastfed babies may be sensitive to something the mother just ate, a condition indicated by an irritated red ring around the rectum. Cow's milk, soy, corn, wheat and eggs are frequent offenders, while flatulence and gas can be caused by the mother eating garlic, onion, beans or cabbage. Dr. Smith recommends that nursing mothers avoid these foods and any others that seem to precipitate colic attacks. Chocolate, alcohol, coffee, spicy foods and excessive quantities of fruit are often cited as colic problems as well.

Traditional treatments for breastfeeding mothers include medicinal strength herbal teas made of **catnip, cinnamon, dill, fennel, lemon balm** and **chamomile**. The teas' soothing properties pass into breast milk and on to the baby's stomach. Weak or diluted teas can be given to babies by the dropperful every 15 minutes. A medicinal strength tea uses 1 tablespoon dried herb per cup of boiling water, steeped for 10 to 15 minutes in a covered container (most leaves and blossoms) or simmered over low heat for 10 to 15 minutes (most roots, barks and seeds). This tea should be diluted with 2 to 3 parts water for direct feeding to infants.

For the treatment of colic, herbalist David Hoffmann recommends "grippe water," an old fashioned infusion of dill seed rarely used in the U.S. even though it's still listed in the *United States Pharmacopeia*. Make your own by pouring 1 cup boiling water over 2 tablespoons **dill seed,** cover and let stand 10 minutes. An equally effective "grippe water" can be made with **fenugreek seed, aniseed, caraway seed** or **fennel seed**. All are aromatic, carminative and relaxing. Like the teas described above, all can be taken by the nursing mother or given directly to the child.

Catnip tea is an important antispasmodic and carminative for children. It combines well with chamomile and any of the seed teas decribed above.

Lemon balm extracts are popular in Europe for treating colic. In addition to brewing lemon balm tea, you may want to make an alcohol-free tincture using vegetable glycerine, which has a sweet taste and is widely used for children's tonics. Cover fresh or dried lemon balm with vegetable glycerine (available from health food stores and herbal tea companies) in a glass jar, cover and let stand in a warm place for several weeks, shaking every few days. Strain and pour into dropper bottles. Give in dropperful doses as needed.

In her *Encyclopedia of Natural Healing for Children and Infants,* Mary Bove recommends applying a fomentation (warm compress) or massage oil containing **lavender, lobelia** or **catnip** to the child's abdomen. To prepare a fomentation, brew an extra strong tea using any of these herbs alone or in combination (2 tablespoons tea per cup of boiling water). Let cool until comfortably warm. Saturate a cloth diaper or small towel with the tea, wring it out just enough to control dripping and apply it to the stomach area. Repeat the procedure every few minutes to keep the area warm or place a hot water bottle over the compress.

Alternatively, make an oil infusion of these herbs by pouring olive oil over loosely packed lavender, lobelia, catnip and/or chamomile and heat over simmering water in a double boiler or in a glass jar placed on a rack in a pan of simmering water for 1 to 2 hours. Strain and pour into amber glass bottles or glass jars, label and store away from heat and light. To help soothe the pain of colic, massage this oil around the stomach area and keep it warm with a warm towel just out of the dryer or a hot water bottle. If using a hot water bottle, protect the child's skin with a layer of toweling and use comfortably hot—not scalding hot—water.

Any relaxing herb (**chamomile, hops, lavender blossoms, lemon balm, skullcap, passionflower** or **lobelia**) can be brewed as a strong tea and added to the baby's bath water for additional antispasmodic therapy. Adding a cup or two of an extra strong fragrant tea to bath water creates a pleasant aromatherapy experience for both child and parent.

Constipation

Sluggish, infrequent bowel movements are almost always caused by insufficient fiber in the diet, dehydration and physical inactivity, though they are sometimes caused by food sensitivities (dairy products are a common culprit), prescription drugs or a physical obstruction. Assuming your bowel is not obstructed, these simple steps might help:

- Drink a large glass of water every hour or two all day long.
- Stir 1 teaspoon to 1 tablespoon of psyllium husk powder, guar gum, pectin or a similar soluble fiber into a glass of water every morning and night.
- As a last resort, take a mild herbal laxative, such as a small amount of **cascara sagrada** or **senna**

Cascara *(Rhamnus purshiana)* is a bitter tonic and one of the oldest, most reliable remedies for chronic constipation. It is not habit forming and helps tone the intestines although, like all laxatives, it should be taken only as needed. Cascara is a common ingrediant in herbal laxatives sold in health food stores and you can brew cascara tea by pouring 1 cup of boiling water over 1 tablespoon shredded bark and letting the infusion stand for 1 hour. Take up to 2 cups daily on an empty stomach until the condition is relieved, which shouldn't take long. Do not use fresh cascara bark; it should have dried for at least 1 year for best results.

American **senna** *(Cassia marilandica)* is a more powerful laxative and can cause cramps or griping unless combined with aromatic herbs such as **ginger** and **chamomile**. To brew senna tea, combine 4 tablespoons senna, 1 teaspoon dried ginger or 1 tablespoon fresh ginger and 2 cups water in a covered pan. Bring just to a boil, then simmer over low heat for 20 to 30 minutes. Remove from heat, add 1 tablespoon dried chamomile blossoms and/or 1 tablespoon fennel seed, replace cover and let stand an additional 10 to 15 minutes. Take in 1/4 cup doses every few hours. Senna usually relieves constipation within 6 to 8 hours. It is not recommended for use during pregnancy or by the elderly.

Another herb that relieves constipation is **yellow dock root** *(Rumex crispus)*. Best known as a tonic for the blood and as a treatment for skin disorders, yellow dock promotes bile production, improves digestion and acts as a mild laxative. To brew yellow dock tea, combine 1 teaspoon herb with 1 cup water, bring to a boil in a covered pan, reduce heat and simmer gently for 10 to 15 minutes, then let stand another 5 to 10 minutes. If desired, add 1 teaspoon of an aromatic herb such as chamomile when you remove the pan from the stove. Drink in 1/4 cup doses throughout the day. Ten drops of yellow dock tincture daily will also prevent constipation.

A dark tar made of boiled **aloe vera** leaves used to be a popular laxative, but this powerful cathartic remedy is no longer aloe vera's claim to fame. Today aloe vera is best known for the soothing gel found in its green and yellow leaves. Its bitter cathartic chemicals are found in the skin of the leaves, which is why plain or clear aloe vera juice or gel does not have a pronounced laxative action. However, capsules containing whole leaf extracts are sold in health food stores and any "whole leaf" aloe vera product will have a laxative effect. These are usually gentle in action (a single capsule will not have a dramatic influence) and can safely be taken in small doses until the condition is relieved.

Arnold Ehret's "intestinal broom" is still famous in health circles nearly 75 years after his death. The recipe, which appears in *Arnold Ehret's Mucusless Diet Healing System* follows:

> Combine 6 parts ground senna leaves, 3 parts ground buckthorn bark and 1 part psyllium seed husks. Mix well. Combine 1/10 part powdered sassafras root bark, ½ part ground dark anise seed, 1/10 part ground buchu leaves, ½ part ground blonde psyllium seed, ⅛ part powdered Irish moss, ⅛ part granulated agar agar and ½ part ground dark fennel seed. Mix well with the first three ingredients.
>
> To use the intestinal broom, take half a teaspoon or less with a glass of water, the recommended daily dose for adults, or adjust as desired.
>
> To brew as a tea, add ½ teaspoon to 1 cup boiling water and let stand 10 to 15 minutes.

Similar blends of constipation-relieving herbs are sold as tablets and teas in health food stores. Look for ingredients such as those listed above for an effective balance of stimulating, cramp-relieving, aromatic herbs. One famous brand, Swiss Kriss, contains **senna, strawberry leaves, peach leaves, anise seed, caraway seed, hibiscus** and **calendula flowers,** a blend that is so fragrant that the loose tea comes with instructions for making a facial steam treatment by pouring boiling water over the herbs and inhaling the steam while covering the head with a large towel. This is one laxative treatment that's as well known as a rejuvenating skin treatment as it is for relieving constipation.

John Lust recommends the juice of ½ lemon in a glass of warm water in the morning to promote healthy bowel movements, followed by 8 ounces fresh raw carrot juice with 8 ounces apple juice, or 6 ounces carrot juice mixed with 5 ounces beet juice and 5 ounces cucumber juice.

Prevent future constipation by drinking large amounts of water and eating more raw fruits and vegetables, dried fruits, whole grains and other whole foods.

Crohn's Disease

With symptoms ranging from debilitating indigestion to chronic and often bloody diarrhea, low fever, weight loss, weakness and colicky pain in the abdomen, Crohn's disease is a terrible affliction. Its complications include abscesses, infected fistulas, perforation of the intestine, gangrenous sores on the body, malnutrition and cancer of the colon. Orthodox treatment includes prednisone and similar drugs and, in severe cases, removal of the large intestine. Most physicians believe the disease is incurable and irreversible.

Opinions about Crohn's disease vary, but many practitioners think it may be caused by an infection, immune disorder or even an inherited defect. Nutritionally oriented physicians believe food allergies and sensitivities are its primary cause.

In April of 1978, Richard Miller, D.D.S. published an article about colitis in *Let's Live* magazine, in which he explained that he had suffered from Crohn's disease for 11 years. His article described the self-help program that had kept him symptom-free for a year, even though when he began that program he was taking 15 mg of prednisone daily to control inflammation, plus four Lomotil for diarrhea, eight Azulfidine for inflammation, and 10 mg Valium to control muscle cramping. In the January 1994 issue of *Let's Live,* he updated his report, noting that he has been symptom-free for 16 years and that a battery of tests done the previous year showed no sign of the disease. Dr. Miller's program emphasizes:

- Improved digestion
- The elimination of white sugar, refined flour, additives, preservatives and allergenic foods
- The supplementation of digestive enzymes
- An alkalizing diet emphasizing fruits and vegetables
- Improved strategies for coping with stress

Dr. Miller publishes a bimonthly newsletter, *GI Health* (3604 Forest Drive, Alexandria, Va. 22302).

Herbs useful in the treatment of Crohn's disease can be taken as teas, tinctures or in capsules, in packaged herbal products or in blends you prepare yourself. Any of the therapies listed for diarrhea, diverticulitis or irritable bowel syndrome are worth trying, although they offer only short term relief from a problem that requires a nutritional overhaul for lasting improvement. **Comfrey** leaf and comfrey root tea (see notes on comfrey's safety, page 38) are especially therapeutic because comfrey contains a cell growth stimulant that speeds the healing of inflamed, irritated or damaged tissue in addition to soothing intestinal surfaces. I agree with Rosemary Gladstar and other herbalists who defend comfrey's safety record and believe that unless a person has a liver disease, it is likely to be far more beneficial than dangerous. A blend containing comfrey and other appropriate herbs should be safe in any quantity; up to 3 or 4 cups of straight comfrey tea per day or 1/2 to 1 teaspoon of comfrey tincture taken twice or three times daily, especially for one to two weeks, should be equally harmless and speed healing.

Slippery elm bark, arrowroot and other gentle sources of soluble fiber can be used in conjunction with or in place of powdered psyllium husks to help prevent both diarrhea and constipation.

The astringent herbs **bayberry bark, witch hazel bark, oak bark** and **cranesbill root** help firm the tissue and reduce discharge and secretions. The carminative herbs **chamomile, angelica, lemon balm, cardamom seed, caraway seed, calamus root, ginger, dill, cayenne pepper** and **peppermint** help relieve gas and flatulence, while the bitter herbs **gentian root, horehound, goldenseal** and **Swedish bitters** improve digestion and the antispasmodic herbs **cramp bark, skullcap, lobelia, valerian** and **wild yam root** help prevent cramping. Look for teas, capsules and tinctures that contain such blends of these herbs. Because Crohn's disease is such a serious illness, it is worth exploring nutritional and herbal strategies with the help of a naturopath, experienced herbalist or other healthcare professional.

Diarrhea

Almost everyone has suffered from diarrhea, but here in the U.S. we don't consider it the life-threatening disorder it is in many countries, where the dehydration it produces can be fatal. To treat diarrhea, take 1 teaspoon to 1 tablespoon **green clay**, the kind sold in health food stores, stirred into a glass of water. Clay has a soothing effect on irritated intestinal lining; it absorbs toxins and helps reverse the condition.

We associate **powdered psyllium husks** with accelerated bowel function because it's usually recommended for those with sluggish elimination, but when the problem is diarrhea, psyllium has the opposite effect: it slows things down by absorbing fluid and by helping create well formed stools. Clay and psyllium can be used together in juice or water. Avoid breathing psyllium husk powder; it can be allergenic. Add between one teaspoon and one tablespoon powdered clay to half a cup of juice, cool tea or water in a covered jar and shake well or, for better results, blend in a blender. Add two teaspoons powdered psyllium husks plus half a cup of water and a pinch of unrefined sea salt and shake well again. Pour into a glass and drink quickly, before the psyllium causes the liquid to gel.

If treatment lasts more than a few days, clay and fiber become a nutritional concern because they may leach minerals from the body. Trace mineral supplements prevent deficiencies if taken between (not with) these treatments.

Arrowroot, Jerusalem artichoke flour and other starches help reduce the amount of fluid lost and restore intestinal flora. William H. Lee recommends a blend of equal parts fresh, raw cabbage and beet juices, equal parts papaya and pineapple juices, or equal parts blackberry and carrot juices. Astringent teas such as **bayberry bark, witch hazel bark, oak bark, princess pine** and **cranesbill** (wild geranium), astringent fruits such as **blackberries** and **blueberries**, **cayenne pepper** in capsules, **grapefruit seed extract** in capsules, large amounts (a dozen or more capsules) of **acidophilus** or similar "friendly bacteria" supplements and large quantities of water with a pinch of unrefined sea salt to prevent dehydration are appropriate therapies. If the diarrhea is likely to be caused by intestinal parasites, use an appropriate anthelmintic (anti-parasite) treatment such as grapefruit seed extract capsules. Take according to package directions to prevent infection or double the recommended dosage to treat an infestation.

Diverticulitis and Colitis

Both disorders are caused by inflammation of the colon. Colitis brings alternating bouts of diarrhea and constipation, while diverticulitis causes intense pain and discomfort. Holistic health practitioners link both disorders to diet: food sensitivities, too little fiber, too much wheat and dairy, too little variety in food choices or, too much cooked and processed food. The long term cure is a complete dietary overhaul in which these factors are addressed.

For short-term relief, fresh vegetable and non-acidic fruit juices provide nutrition without irritating intestinal lining. Demulcent, mucilaginous herbs like **comfrey root, slippery elm bark** and **arrowroot** soothe and nourish. Add between 1 and 3 teaspoons of powdered root or bark to a glass of water, stir well and drink. Eliminate foods most likely to cause intestinal irritation, such as wheat, dairy products and caffeine. Add water soluble fiber to the diet, such as psyllium husk powder or pectin. Drink several glasses of water in addition to herbal teas and juices; avoid coffee, colas and alcoholic beverages for now.

In the May 1992 issue of *Let's Live*, Jonathan Wright, M.D., described his treatment of ulcerative colitis. He associated this disorder with a history of chronic ear infections, asthma or hay fever and attributed the disease to untreated food allergies. According to Wright, more than two-thirds of ulcerative colitis patients have incompletely digested food in the stool, small particles of which can be absorbed into the body (this disorder is called "leaky gut syndrome") causing further allergic reactions. Wright's therapy for ulcerative colitis includes testing for food allergies, stomach function, pancreas function and intestinal bacteria, then supplying supplements as needed. Patients with advanced cases often have insufficient hydrochloric acid, digestive enzymes and beneficial bacteria and their diets emphasize the foods they are most allergic or sensitive to. Vitamin and mineral deficiencies are common and require supplementation.

To prevent deficiencies of this type, consider adding digestive enzymes, hydrochloric acid, acidophilus supplements, vitamins and minerals to your diet in addition to keeping a food diary and avoiding foods that seem to make the problem worse. Researchers in the U. S. and Europe repeatedly find that cow's milk dairy products, coffee, strong black tea, alcohol and the gluten found in wheat, oats, barley and rye are common offenders.

Remember that plain drinking water is a cure for many digestive and intestinal problems. If you aren't already doing so, try to drink up to a gallon of water daily, adding a pinch of unrefined sea salt to each glass.

Psyllium husks, described in the preceding section as a treatment for diarrhea, can help stabilize the unpredictable bouts of diarrhea and constipation by absorbing liquid, forming well shaped stools and encouraging regular bowel movements. Drinking extra water is important whenever you take psyllium.

The herbalist Richard Mabey recommends brewing the following tea for colitis:

> Combine 1 part wild yam root, 1 part goldenseal, 1/2 part calamus root and 3 parts marshmallow root. Add 1 tablespoon of this blend to 2 cups water in a covered pan, bring it to a boil, lower the heat and simmer gently for 10 to 15 minutes and remove from heat. Add 1 teaspoon chamomile, cover and let stand an additional 10 minutes. Drink up to 4 cups daily, as desired, until the problem subsides.

Gas, Flatulence

Intestinal gas or "wind" can be caused by eating too fast, swallowing air, eating gas-producing foods such as beans, drinking carbonated beverages, chewing gum, talking with your mouth full or eating dairy products if you are lactose intolerant. In addition to the digestive enzymes Beano and Lactaid (see pages 17 and 12), look to the carminative herbs for relief: **angelica root, aniseed, caraway seed, cardamom seed, catnip, cayenne pepper, celery seed, chamomile, cinnamon, cloves, fennel seed, ginger, lemon balm, licorice root, peppermint, spearmint** and **Swedish bitters**. The herbs listed above can be taken as teas or tinctures, alone or in combination. Seeds, roots and barks should be brewed as decoctions (1 teaspoon to 1 tablespoon herb simmered in 1 cup water for 10 to 15 minutes) while leaves and blossoms should be brewed as infusions (1 teaspoon to 1 tablespoon herb per cup of boiling water, steeped for 10 to 15 minutes). A teaspoon of herb makes a beverage strength tea; a tablespoon makes a medicinal strength tea.

To make your own effective tincture, cover any or all of the above herbs (any quantity or combination) with alcohol, vegetable glycerine or cider vinegar in a glass jar. Alcohol (vodka, rum, brandy, etc.) is the preferred liquid because it dissolves most plant constituents and the resulting tinctures have an indefinite shelf life, but vegetable glycerine and cider vinegar make effective tinctures for those who prefer not to use alcohol.

Leave the glass jar in a warm place for at least a month, shaking it every few days. Strain and store the tincture in amber glass bottles away from heat and light.

One of Germany's best selling cures for abdominal distress is a tincture of lemon balm *(Melissa officinalis)*; similar "melissa waters" are popular throughout Europe. To relieve flatulance, take at least 1 teaspoon of any carminative tincture with a glass of water every half hour until symptoms subside.

In severe cases, take two capsules containing activated charcoal with a glass of water every 20 minutes until symptoms subside. To prevent flatulence:

- Take Swedish bitters before eating
- Eat slowly and chew food well
- Avoid carbonated beverages and foods that don't agree with you
- Take hydrochloric acid supplements or digestive enzymes as needed
- Supplement your diet with acidophilus and other friendly bacteria
- Avoid stress while eating

Gastritis

Inflammation of the stomach's lining can cause short-term discomfort or chronic pain. If it doesn't go away quickly in response to the clearing of an infection or reactions to specific foods, the cause may be any of the following irritants: food that is too hot or too cold, food that contains chemical irritants (alcohol, spices, curries, greasy foods, vinegar) or mechanical irritants (insoluble fiber, such as wheat bran).

To repair the problem avoid the above as well as tobacco, drink fresh, raw juices and take demulcent or soothing herbs such as **comfrey root, marshmallow root** and **chamomile** in teas or tinctures. One soothing tea blend consists of 1 part comfrey root, 1 part marshmallow root and 1 part slippery elm bark simmered as a decoction (2 cups water to 2 tablespoons tea, cooked over low heat for 10 to 15 minutes). For added benefits, add a teaspoon of chamomile when you take the pan off the stove and let the tea stand, covered, an additional 10 minutes. Drink as often as desired.

Remember to drink as much water as possible during gastritis attacks, starting with 8-ounce glasses every 30 to 40 minutes until symptoms subside. If desired, add up to a tablespoon of powdered comfrey root, marshmallow root, slippery elm bark, arrowroot or a similar demulcent starch to the water just before drinking.

In addition, review the suggestions for treating ulcers, since peptic ulcers and gastritis usually respond to the same therapies.

Heartburn

Heartburn has nothing to do with the heart but was named for the approximate location of burning pain that occurs when stomach acid leaks into the esophagus. This often happens when people overeat or eat foods that are too spicy or too greasy. Common offenders include chocolate, caffeine, onions, tomatoes, citrus fruits and peppery sausages. A Mayo Clinic survey of 1500 patients concluded that alcohol, smoking, aspirin and nonsteroidal anti-inflammatory drugs, all of which are considered risk factors for gastroesophageal reflux disease, are in fact not important. The primary risk factor found in the survey was obesity. If you are overweight and suffer from heartburn, losing the excess pounds will probably remove this unpleasant symptom.

To alleviate heartburn, drink an 8-ounce glass of water every 20 to 30 minutes until pain subsides, drink a cup of **licorice root** tea or take 100 grams de-glycyrrhinized licorice, take any **angelica** product according to label directions or take 1 teaspoon to 1 tablespoon of **lemon balm** (melissa) tincture. Prevent this condition by eating small meals often rather than large meals infrequently, avoid eating late at night, avoid foods that are overspiced, greasy, sugary or acidic, take Swedish bitters before eating, take digestive supplements as needed, experiment with the basic rules of food combining (don't eat fruit after a dinner of protein and carbohydrates, for example) and take an acidophilus supplement daily.

Drugs that relax smooth muscles, such as the asthma drug theophylline, contribute to the problem because heartburn occurs when the esophageal sphincter muscle relaxes and allows stomach acid and pepsin to enter the esophagus. Like theophylline, the essential oil of peppermint causes the esophageal sphincter to relax, allowing digestive juices to leak into the esophagus, which makes heartburn worse. Although peppermint is highly regarded for other types of indigestion, its essential oil is not recommended for heartburn. Peppermint leaf tea is less concentrated and less likely to cause this reaction.

Aside from peppermint oil, all of the carminative herbs are effective treatments, especially **lemon balm**, **dill**, **chamomile** and **aniseed**. For best results, take up to a teaspoon of tincture or a cup of medicinal strength tea (1 tablespoon herb per cup of water) and repeat every hour until symptoms subside. Swedish bitters can be taken before and after eating and again when heartburn symptoms appear to prevent and treat this condition.

Hemorrhoids

Hemorrhoids, or piles, are painful varicose veins in the rectum or anus. Their most common cause is chronic constipation, often associated with a lack of exercise. They are also common during pregnancy. To help relieve hemorrhoid symptoms, drink more water and fluids, increase soluble fibers in the diet, such as **powdered psyllium husks, slippery elm bark** and **pectin,** improve nutrition with raw juices and whole fruits and vegetables, take a tablespoon of cold pressed flaxseed oil daily and move bowels promptly instead of suppressing their movements. Hemorrhoids are a risk factor in sedentary occupations, so be sure to get plenty of active excercise.

For relief from pain, apply **aloe vera gel** or any strong astringent tea such as **bayberry bark, witch hazel bark, oak bark,** or **cranesbill root** to the affected area several times daily. To brew any of these teas for use as a wash or compress, combine 1 cup water with 1 tablespoon herbs and simmer in a covered pan for 15 to 20 minutes. Remove from heat and let stand until cool. Refrigerate for best results as cold causes the veins to contract. Apply cold tea with a cloth or paper towel and hold it in place for as long as possible.

The same astringent teas can be taken internally to help treat the problem from the inside out. Astringent fruits or juices may be more to your liking as the teas described here do not taste pleasant. Blackberries and blackberry juice are beneficial and can be taken in any form and quantity.

In addition to the thereapies described above, Rosemary Gladstar recommends applying a poultice made of water or witch hazel extract (the kind sold in pharmacies as a skin care product) and green clay. Add just enough liquid to form a thick paste and apply it directly to the hemmorrhoids, then leave it in place until it's completely dry. Remove the clay in the bathtub or shower.

Indigestion, Dyspepsia

This catch-all diagnosis covers a variety of symptoms ranging from simple discomfort to heartburn, pain and flatulence. It can be caused by irregular meals (the digestive tract loves a dependable schedule), overeating, eating too fast and eating the wrong foods. For immediate relief, David Hoffmann recommends **meadowsweet tea,** which settles the stomach and reduces acidity, **Irish moss** and other demulcents, bitter herbs before or after eating to stimulate digestion and carminatives like **aniseed, lemon balm, cardamom, fennel** and **peppermint** to relieve gas. Follow the standard recipes for making teas: use 1 teaspoon dried herb per cup of water for a beverage strength tea and 1 tablespoon per cup for medicinal strength; infuse leaves and blossoms in boiling water for 10 to 15 minutes in a teapot or capped glass jar and decoc roots, bark and seeds by simmering them in a covered pan for 10 to 15 minutes over low heat. Drink up to 4 cups of any of the teas listed above per day, or take 1/2 to 1 teaspoon tincture 3 to 4 times daily.

Another sensible strategy is to take a teaspoon to a tablespoon of **Swedish bitters** or a similar bitter aperitif before eating. The bitter taste stimulates saliva, bile production and the secretion of other digestive juices. You may want to experiment with hydrochloric acid (HCl) supplements and digestive enzymes as well. Because indigestion is so often linked to food sensitivities, keep a food diary and eliminate whatever doesn't agree with you from your diet. Last, drink more water, especially when pain occurs, up to one 8-ounce glass every 15 to 20 minutes until pain subsides.

See also the descriptions of gas/flatulence and gastritis.

Irritable Bowel Syndrome

IBS is a chronic disorder in which the muscle of the lower colon produces exaggerated contractions, causing pain, gas, bloating, and alternating constipation and diarrhea. The cause may be food sensitivities, a lack of dietary fiber, insufficient beneficial bacteria or stress.

All of the recommendations for treating diverticulitis, colitis, Crohn's disease and diarrhea apply here; refer to those sections for specific instructions.

In general, drink frequent glasses of water, gradually increase the amount of soluble fiber in your diet, drink raw fruit and vegetable juices and treat constipation with mild laxative herbs (**senna** or **cascara sagrada** as recommended in the section describing constipation). Avoid common allergens and work toward a more tranquil life.

In addition to the herbs recommended for diverticulitis, colitis, Crohn's disease and constipation, consider the lowly **dandelion**. Dandelion leaves and root are both therapeutic. A tonic to the liver and the entire digestive tract, dandelion is a bitter herb that is high in potash and inulin, a carbohydrate that is so easily assimilated, it is recommended for the nutritional support of diabetics. Fresh dandelion leaves in salad, dandelion leaf tea (infusion) and dendelion root tea (decoction) all benefit people with colitis, hepatitis, indigestion, irritable bowel syndrome and other digestive problems. Use 1 to 3 teaspoons dried herb per cup of water to brew dandelion tea. This herb combines well with other herbs, especially **ginger root** and **licorice root**. For a combination tea, blend equal parts of these dried roots and simmer 1 tablespoon herb in 2 cups water for 15 minutes. Drink as much of the tea as often as desired.

Ulcers

Ulcers don't just happen, they are caused by factors that need correcting even after herbs relieve their pain. Try avoiding common allergens like dairy products. Identify foods that don't agree with you, which probably include foods high in acid. Don't take digestive enzymes. Reduce the stress in your life and improve your nutrition. Drink fresh, raw juices as much as possible, especially **cabbage juice**, which Europeans consider a specific for ulcers. One quart per day for a week literally cures most ulcers, which a friend found hard to believe until I showed her medical reports substantiating this claim. She had been hospitalized for a bleeding ulcer once before, so she recognized the symptoms as soon as they appeared. Two days and two quarts of green cabbage juice later, she was tired of the taste but exclaimed she had never felt better. That was three years ago and her ulcer has not returned.

Another specific for ulcers is **licorice root**. Use any licorice root preparation for short periods; for therapy lasting more than one week, take de-glycyrrhinized licorice root tablets (chew before swallowing for best results) to prevent the fluid retention and elevated blood pressure associated with untreated licorice root.

Although many physicians recommend a bland diet with no spicy foods, **cayenne pepper** capsules, the hotter the better, are more likely to help, especially when bleeding is a factor. If you are taking cayenne capsules for the first time, be sure to swallow them with plenty of food and water. If you experience a sensation similar to heartburn within an hour of taking cayenne, drink apple juice or peppermint tea. The sensation is not heartburn—and it isn't your ulcer—but rather a reaction to the peppers. Because cayenne pepper decreases sensitivity to pain the more often it is taken, this short-lived side effect doesn't recur if you remember to take 1 or 2 capsules twice or three times daily. Cayenne is a catalyst herb, meaning that it improves the effectiveness of other herbs by increasing circulation and digestive activity. Take a cayenne pepper capsule with any medicinal tea and you will speed and increase its benefits.

Comfrey root and other mucilaginous herbs, like **slippery elm bark** and **arrowroot,** soothe damaged tissue. A tablespoon of any of these powdered herbs can be added to a glass of water and stirred well before drinking to coat the stomach, relieve pain and strengthen the system.

Two ounces (1/4 cup) **aloe vera gel** or juice taken three times daily is another effective ulcer treatment. Whole aloe vera leaf is a cathartic laxative, but the inner gel of the succulent leaf does not contain any bitter cathartic ingredients. This inner gel is sold as aloe vera juice and aloe vera gel in health food stores. The English herbalist David Hoffmann does not recommend aloe vera to pregnant women or nursing mothers, but it is otherwise recognized as safe. Check labels for suggested dosages and to be sure the product does not contain chemical preservatives or ingredients other than cold process aloe vera gel from the plant's inner leaf.

SUMMARY: TWELVE STEPS TO BETTER DIGESTION

1. Eat something raw before you eat something cooked.
2. Take Swedish bitters or any bitter herb or aperitif, holding it in your mouth to activate the taste buds, before eating.
3. Allow time for relaxed eating. Make mealtimes pleasant. Focus on soothing music and the tastes you're experiencing; avoid arguments and other disruptions.
4. Chew every mouthful carefully. Some nutritionists recommend chewing each bite at least 30 or 50 or even a hundred times. Start with 10 or 15.
5. Eat more raw food. If you can't eat a vegetable raw, cook it lightly or slowly. Replace frying, boiling, and pressure cooking with light steaming or poaching.
6. Drink fresh, raw vegetable or fruit juice every day.
7. Drink 2 to 4 quarts of water between meals.
8. Eat a variety of foods from different food families.
9. Avoid common allergens, or test yourself for specific food sensitivities and avoid those foods.
10. Take digestive enzymes and/or hydrochloric acid with meals to aid digestion (not recommended for ulcer patients).

11. Take acidophilus supplements daily.
12. Spend at least 20 minutes in active exercise, practice deep breathing and lie on a slant board or practice an inverted yoga posture every day.
13. Enjoy life!

RECOMMENDED READING AND RESOURCES

Herbals

Foster, Steven, and James A. Duke. *Peterson Field Guides: Eastern/Central Medicinal Plants*. Boston: Houghton Mifflin, 1990. Superior field guide with well documented medicinal uses.

Gladstar, Rosemary. *Herbal Healing for Women*. New York: Fireside, Simon & Schuster, 1993. Exciting herbal alternatives for all female disorders, including indigestion, ulcers and related illnesses.

Hoffmann, David. *The Holistic Herbal*. Dorset, England: Element Books, 1983. Popular modern reference.

Keville, Kathi. *The Illustrated Herbal Encyclopedia*. New York: Bantam Doubleday, 1992. Recommended.

Kloss, Jethro. *Back to Eden*. Loma Linda, Calif.: Back to Eden Books, 1988. Updated classic, belongs in everyone's library.

Lust, John. *The Herb Book*. New York: Bantam Books, 1974. Excellent, inexpensive basic herbal.

Reader's Digest. *Magic and Medicine of Plants*. Pleasantville, N.Y.: Reader's Digest Association, 1986. Good overview, some overly cautious warnings.

Theiss, Barbara and Peter. *The Family Herbal*. Rochester, Vt.: Healing Arts Press, 1989. Introduction to European herbalism, recommended.

Tierra, Michael. *The Way of Herbs*. New York: Pocket Books, 1983. Recommended basic herbal.

Weiss, Rodolf Fritz. *Herbal Medicine*. English translation of the sixth German edition, 1988. Imported by Medicina Biologica, Portland, Oreg. Excellent reference.

Organizations

American Botanical Council, P. O. Box 201660, Austin, Tex. 78720.

American Herb Association, P. O. Box 1673, Nevada City, Calif. 95959.

Herb Research Foundation, 1007 Pearl Street, Suite 200, Boulder, Colo. 80302.

Northeast Herbal Association, P. O. Box 479, Milton, N.Y. 12547.

Magazines

The Herb Companion, 201 East 4th Street, Loveland, Colo. 80537.

The Herb Quarterly, P. O. Box 689, San Anselmo, Calif. 94960.

HerbalGram, P. O. Box 201660, Austin, Tex. 78720.

Herbal Education

Directory of Herbal Education, Intra-American Specialties, 3014 North 400 West, West Lafayette, Ind. 47906. Review of on-site and correspondence courses.

East West Master Course in Herbology by Michael Tierra, P. O. Box 712, Santa Cruz, Calif. 95061.

The Science and Art of Herbalism: A Home Study Course by Rosemary Gladstar, P. O. Box 420, East Barre, Vt. 05649.

Dried Herbs and Teas

Avena Botanicals, P. O. Box 365, West Rockport, Me. 04865.

Blessed Herbs, 109 Barre Plains Road, Oakham, Me. 01068.

Frontier Cooperative Herbs, P. O. Box 299, Norway, Ia. 52318.

Green Terrestrial, P. O. Box 41, Route 9W, Milton, N.Y. 12547.
The Herb Closet, 104 Main Street, Montpelier, Vt. 05602.
The Herbfarm, 32804 Issaquah Fall City Road, Fall City, Wash. 98024.
Island Herbs, Ryan Drum, Waldron Island, Wash. 98297.
Jean's Greens, 54 McManus Road, Rensselaerville, N.Y. 12147.
Mountain Rose Herbs, Box 2000, Redway, Calif. 95560.
Pacific Botanicals, Catalog Request, 4350 Fish Hatchery Road, Grants Pass, Oreg. 97527.
Sage Mountain Herb Products, P. O. Box 420, East Barre, Vt. 05649.
Trinity Herbs, P. O. Box 199, Bodega, Calif. 94992.
Wild Weeds, P. O. Box 88, Redway, Calif. 95560.

Index